P9-DMS-385

DATE DUE

NOV 1 2 1997			
NOV - 7 1997			
GAYLORD			PRINTED IN U.S.A.

Pictorial Human
Embryology

Nature's Rudiments and Attempts are involved in obscurity and deep night, and so perplext with sub-tilties, that they delude the most piercing wit, as well as the sharpest eye. Nor can we easier discover the secret recesses, and dark principles of Generation than the method of the fabrick and composure of the whole world. In this reciprocal interchange of Generation and Corruption consists the Eternity and Duration of mortal creatures. And as the Rising and setting of the Sun, doth by continued revolutions complete and perfect time; so doth the alternative vicissitude of Individuums, by a constant repetition of the same species, perpetuate the continuance of fading things.

William Harvey, *Anatomical Exercitations Concerning the Generation of Living Creatures* (London, 1653), ex. XIV

PICTORIAL
HUMAN
EMBRYOLOGY

Illustrations and text
by Stephen G. Gilbert

UNIVERSITY OF WASHINGTON PRESS

Seattle and London

For my father,

who showed me where to find frog's eggs

By the same author:

Pictorial Anatomy of the Necturus

Pictorial Anatomy of the Cat

Pictorial Anatomy of the Frog

Pictorial Anatomy of the Fetal Pig

Pictorial Anatomy of the Dogfish

Atlas of General Zoology

Copyright © 1989 by the University of Washington Press
Printed in the United States of America

Library of Congress Cataloging-in-Publication Data
Gilbert, Stephen G.
    Pictorial human embryology. Illustrations and text by
Stephen G. Gilbert.
    Bibliography: p.
    1. Embryology, Human—Atlases. I. Title.
QM602.G55   611'.013'0222   87-34642
ISBN 0-295-96631-9 (cl.)
ISBN 0-295-96632-7 (pb.)

Contents

Preface

Pictorial Human Embryology is designed for
students of medicine and allied health sciences
who study embryology in connection with
human anatomy. For them it will serve as an
outline and reference which will supplement
lectures and texts. It may also be of interest to
students of biology, zoology, and comparative
anatomy.

The use of atlases to supplement textbooks of
anatomy has long been widely accepted, but in
the case of embryology there are few such atlases, and those currently available are for the
most part laboratory manuals designed to facil-
itate the identification of structures seen in
photomicrographs of sectioned embryos. In
contrast to this approach I have illustrated the
development of each system as a whole, from
its earliest appearance to the end of the embryonic period, as a sequence of related drawings;
a student can observe the origin, development,
and transformation of embryonic structures by
following them from one illustration to the
next. It is my hope that *Pictorial Human Embryology* will enable the student to gain a pan-
oramic view of embryonic development, and
that this view will make lectures and conven-
tional textbook accounts more interesting and
more accessible.

STEPHEN G. GILBERT
Associate Professor
Department of Art as Applied to Medicine
Faculty of Medicine
University of Toronto
Canada

Acknowledgments

I am grateful to Professor Emeritus Nancy Joy and to Professor Linda Wilson-Pauwels, Acting Chair, both of the Department of Art as Applied to Medicine at the University of Toronto, for their support and encouragement during the preparation of this work. I am also grateful to the students in the School of Medical Illustration at the University of Toronto, who pointed out numerous errors and inconsistencies while the work was in progress.

I would like to thank the following individuals: Anne Gilbert, who proofed the galleys; Dave Mazierski, who helped with the layouts; Keith Scott, who gave advice on design; Roy Pearson, who assisted in the preparation of the bibliography; Jeannette Poulin, who made many of the color separations; Ranice Crosby, Steve Toussaint, Professor Anne Agur, Dr. Donald R. Cahill, Dr. Pat Farquharson, and Karen Visser, who read portions of the work and made a number of helpful suggestions.

I would also like to thank Dr. Bruce Fraser of the Faculty of Medicine, Memorial University of Newfoundland, who very generously read and criticized the manuscript. His comments were extremely helpful.

Dr. Michael Wiley of the Faculty of Medicine, University of Toronto, acted as consultant and critic throughout the preparation of the text and illustrations. I am greatly indebted to him for his generous contribution of time and energy.

The illustrations in this book are based on material which appeared in scientific books and journals between 1885 and 1960, during which time the bulk of the literature on human organogenesis was written. Each caption includes a series of numbers in parentheses; these numbers identify the items in the bibliography on which the illustration is based. Major sources are indicated in boldface; other numbers are supplementary sources.

In preparing these illustrations I have drawn on the work of many artists, but first of all I must acknowledge my great indebtedness to James Didusch. The following illustrations are based on his work which appeared in the *Carnegie Contributions to Embryology:* Figures 1–5 (the first three weeks), Figures 17–21 (the early development of the urogenital system); Figures 28, 29, 31, 32, 34, 35 (the early development of the heart); Figures 56, 59, 62, 65 (ventral views of the aortic arches); and Figures 107 and 108 (lateral views of the skull). In addition, many of the marginal diagrams which accompany the text are based on his work.

My illustrations of the cranial nerves and the arteries and veins of the head are based on the work of Dorcas H. Padget. These include: Figures 7–11 (overview of the second month); Figures 57, 60, 63, 66, 69, 72 (cranial arteries); Figures 73–76 (cranial veins); and Figures 89, 91, 93, 95 (cranial nerves).

Max Broedel's illustrations of the development of the kidneys (109) and of the gut (85) were a great source of inspiration. In most of my illustrations I have adopted his method of showing a consecutive series of lateral views, and his inclusion of a small marginal drawing of the embryo to scale.

I have frequently consulted Gasser (1975 [8]) and Blechschmidt (1963 {3}). My Figure 87a is a copy of a drawing by Don Alvarado (fig. 4.1 in Gasser 1975) and is used here by permission of Harper and Row.

I have also found Bradley M. Patten's text and illustrations (4, 5) extremely helpful. Of particular interest are his drawings of the embryonic heart, which are based on his own reconstructions of embryonic pig hearts and on the classic reconstructions of Born (1889 [120]) and Tandler (1912 [133], 1913 [134]). My Figures 39, 43, 51, 53, and 114 are based on Patten's illustrations and are used here by permission of the McGraw-Hill Book Company.

In addition to the individuals mentioned above, I have drawn on the work of many lesser known and anonymous illustrators whose drawings are reproduced in the papers and books listed in the bibliography. Going through this material has made me aware of the enormous debt we owe to the many researchers who have studied individual problems in embryology. This debt can easily be overlooked when we read a concise account of the development of an organ or a system in a current text. We stand not on the shoulders of giants, but on the shoulders of thousands of men and women like ourselves, who found the early stages of human development beautiful and fascinating and mysterious.

Introduction:
Embryos and Illustrators

The first detailed, systematic illustrations based on reconstructions of human embryos were made by Wilhelm His (1831–1904) and published in his classic *Anatomie Menschlicher Embryonen* (Leipzig: F. C. W. Vogel, 1885 [13]). In 1872 His was appointed to the chair of anatomy at the University of Leipzig. There he built a new laboratory and hired a staff which included artists, photographers, technicians, and a sculptor. He also perfected a microtome which, together with new techniques of embedding and staining, made it possible to cut sections thinner and more perfect than any which had been made before.

Previous studies of human embryos had been for the most part based on crudely cut, isolated sections which were sometimes haphazardly compared with other sections from older or younger embryos. An original and outstanding feature of His's work was that he portrayed the whole embryo by making a series of sections arranged in order. He then made graphic reconstructions of individual organs and systems by enlarging and projecting serial sections onto ruled paper. His work was of such outstanding quality that his illustrations are still reproduced in current textbooks.

One of the illustrators employed by His was a young art student named Max Broedel (1870–1941), who was trying to finance his education at the Leipzig Academy of Fine Art by doing technical illustration in his spare time. In addition to his work for His, Broedel was engaged to make illustrations for other prominent anatomists such as Christian Braune and Werner Spalteholz, and he was later employed by Carl Ludwig in the Physiological Institute of the University of Leipzig. It was there that he met the American anatomist Dr. Franklin P. Mall, who was associated with The Johns Hopkins University Medical School and Hospi-tal in Baltimore, Maryland. Mall greatly admired Broedel's work and suggested that he come to the United States.

On January 18, 1884, Broedel arrived in Baltimore and was engaged by Dr. Howard A. Kelly, then chief of gynecology at the Johns Hopkins Hospital, to illustrate his book *Operative Gynecology* (D. Appleton and Company, 1898). This early work established Kelly as the leading American gynecologist, and Broedel's superb illustrations marked a turning point in the history of medical illustration.

At the time of Broedel's arrival in the United States most medical books were illustrated by self-taught technical draughtsmen who were capable only of making uninspired diagrams. Broedel's training in the classical traditions of nineteenth-century draughtsmanship and later, in preclinical medical sciences, enabled him to develop a completely original style which combined scientific accuracy with outstanding artistry.

Most of Broedel's illustrations were in the fields of gynecology and urology. During the course of this work he did two series of embryological drawings which set new standards of excellence and are still considered classics today. They are his illustrations for Kelly and Burnam's 1922 *Diseases of the Kidneys, Ureters, and Bladder* (109) and for Cullen's 1916 *Embryology, Anatomy, and Diseases of the Umbilicus* (85).

In 1910 Thomas Cullen conceived the idea of founding a school of medical illustration as part of The Johns Hopkins University School of Medicine. Henry Walters, a Baltimore businessman and patron of the arts, generously endowed the school, and in 1911 the Department of Art as Applied to Medicine was created with Max Broedel as its first director. It was the first school devoted exclusively to the teaching of medical illustration. Over a period of thirty years, Broedel trained more than two hundred illustrators.

Broedel's first student was James Didusch (1890–1955), who became one of the most accomplished medical illustrators of his day. Didusch was the first employee hired by the newly formed Department of Embryology of the Carnegie Institution of Washington, which was then located in Baltimore and closely associated with The Johns Hopkins University School of Medicine.

During forty-two years with the Carnegie Institution, Didusch illustrated many classics of descriptive embryology written by such eminent embryologists as Franklin P. Mall, George L. Streeter, George W. Corner, and their colleagues. He is responsible for the great majority of the superb illustrations in the *Carnegie Contributions to Embryology,* and his work is widely reproduced in current texts. He was the only one of Broedel's students who devoted most of his working life to embryology, and his contribution to embryological research is unique.

Another of Broedel's students who made a significant contribution to embryology was Dorcas Hager Padget (1906–1973). For many years she assisted Broedel in his teaching, and from 1946 to 1951 she was a research fellow in the Department of Embryology of the Carnegie Institution. During this time she wrote and illustrated the definitive papers on the embryology of the arteries and veins of the head (143, 153, 154). Her reconstructions and illustrations are the most accurate and comprehensive ever done on this subject, and are also of great value for their treatment of the brain and cranial nerves.

Definitive studies on the development of the skeletal and muscular systems (220, 221, 224) were illustrated by Ruth Huntington, who was one of Broedel's colleagues, and who later became his wife. Many other students of Max Broedel contributed illustrations to embryological research. Some of his students founded teaching programs of their own, and the influence of his high standards and unique methods is still felt today. In the words of Thomas S. Cullen, "he revolutionized medical illustration and placed it on a very high plane. His pioneer work . . . has already been of inestimable value to medicine and surgery, and the appreciation of his remarkable contribution will grow greater and greater as the years go by."

The Carnegie Stages

In much of the older embryological literature it was customary to classify an embryo according to either its height or its age in days since fertilization. Such designations were, however, often unsatisfactory. Embryos of any age may vary in height, and fertilization age can seldom be determined exactly. In an effort to address this problem, George L. Streeter surveyed the embryos of the Carnegie Collection. Between 1942 and 1951 he published a series of papers

Table 1. Developmental Stages in Human Embryos

Carnegie Stage	Pairs of somites	Length (mm)	Age (days)	Weeks
1 2 3 4			1.5–3 4 5–6	1
5 { 5a 5b 5c 6 } 6a } 6 6b		0.1–0.2 { 0.1 0.1 0.15–0.2 0.2	7–12 { 7–8 9 11–12 13	2
7 8 9	 1–3	0.4 1.0–1.5 1.5–2.5	16 18 20	3
10 11 12 13	4–12 13–20 21–29 30–?	2–3.5 2.5–4.5 3–5 4–6	22 24 26 28	4
14 15	30–?	5–7 7–9	32 33	5
16 17		8–11 11–14	37 41	6
18 19		13–17 16–18	44 47	7
20 21 22 23		18–22 22–24 23–28 27–31	50 52 54 56	8

titled "Developmental Horizons in Human Embryos" (60, 61, 62, 63), in which he correlated age, height, and development. More recently Ronan O'Rahilly, the present director of the Department of Embryology of the Carnegie Institution, has revised Streeter's work. The following table is adapted from O'Rahilly 1973 (82).

Pictorial Human
Embryology

The First Three Weeks

Fertilization, cleavage, and the morula

Fertilization normally occurs in the distal end
of the uterine tube. At the time of fertilization
the ovum is enclosed in a clear acellular layer
termed the *zona pellucida*, which is thought to
play a role in preventing more than one sper-
matozoon from entering the ovum. The process
of fertilization probably takes a little more than
twenty-four hours. It begins when a spermato-
zoon makes contact with the zona pellucida and
ends with the union of the male and female
pronuclei and the intermingling of maternal
and paternal chromosomes. The fertilized ovum
is then termed a *zygote.*

As the process of fertilization is being completed, the zygote begins to undergo the first of
a series of mitotic divisions termed *cleavage.*
The cells resulting from these divisions are
termed *blastomeres.* As cleavage continues the
blastomeres pass down the uterine tube toward
the uterine cavity, completing the journey in
about three or four days. By the time they
reach the uterine cavity the number of blastomeres has increased to about sixteen and they
form a spherical mass termed a *morula.*

The blastocyst

About the time the morula enters the uterine cavity, a fluid-filled space termed the
blastocoele develops within it, and the mass of
cells as a whole is then termed a *blastocyst.* The
spherical outer wall of the blastocyst is termed
the *trophoblast.* Attached eccentrically to the inner surface of the trophoblast is a cluster of
cells termed the *inner cell mass.*

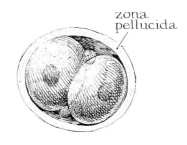

Stage 2   Two blastomeres (82)

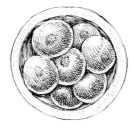

Stage 2   Eight blastomeres (82)

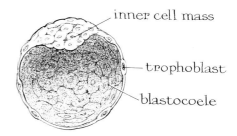

Stage 3   Section of blastocyst (11, 82)

Implantation

About six days after fertilization the zona pellucida degenerates and the blastocyst becomes attached to and embedded in the endometrium. By the eleventh or twelfth day the blastocyst is completely embedded in the endometrium and the defect caused by its entrance is closing (see Figs. 1 and 2).

The trophoblast forms most of the chorion. Its further development is summarized on page 13. The inner cell mass gives rise to the embryo. Its development is described below.

The bilaminar embryonic disc

About the time of implantation the inner cell mass differentiates into two layers termed the *epiblast* and the *hypoblast,* which together constitute the *bilaminar embryonic disc.* At the same time a space termed the *amniotic cavity* develops between the epiblast and the trophoblast. Peripherally the epiblast is continuous with a layer of cells termed amnioblasts, which line the amniotic cavity. As the amniotic cavity is developing, the *primary yolk sac* makes its appearance as a thin layer of cells *(Heuser's membrane)* which forms around the inner surface of the trophoblast (see Figs. 1 and 2).

The secondary yolk sac

Toward the end of the second week (stage 6) a part of the primary yolk sac becomes pinched off and degenerates. The remaining part of the original primary yolk sac is then termed the *secondary yolk sac.* In embryos older than two weeks, the secondary yolk sac is termed simply "the yolk sac."

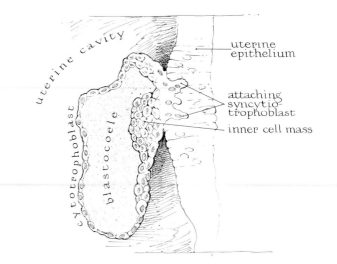
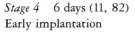

Stage 4 6 days (11, 82)
Early implantation

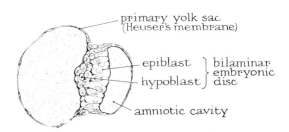

Stage 5c 11 days (36, 79)
Section of bilaminar embryonic disc

Extra-embryonic mesoderm and extra-embryonic coelom

As implantation proceeds an area of tissue termed *extra-embryonic mesoderm* develops between the primary yolk sac and the trophoblast. About the twelfth day (stage 5) vacuoles develop within the extra-embryonic mesoderm. These vacuoles rapidly grow larger and fuse, forming a space termed the *extra-embryonic coelom* (later termed the *chorionic cavity*). The extra-embryonic mesoderm then consists of two layers: one layer (termed *extra-embryonic somatic mesoderm*) lines the trophoblast and the amnion, and the other layer (termed *extra-embryonic splanchnic mesoderm*) covers the secondary yolk sac. The extra-embryonic mesoderm contributes to the formation of the fetal membranes but plays no part in the development of the embryo itself (see Fig. 3).

The trilaminar embryonic disc

About the end of the second week an area of cellular activity termed the *primitive streak* appears in the midline. Certain cells originating in the epiblast converge toward the primitive streak, enter it, and migrate first toward the hypoblast and then laterally and cranially. This process is termed *gastrulation.*

After gastrulation the embryonic disc consists of three layers. (1) The dorsal layer is termed *ectoderm.* It consists of cells which originate in and remain in the epiblast. (2) The middle layer is termed the *intra-embryonic mesoderm.* It consists for the most part of cells which originate in the epiblast and migrate inward to take up a position between the hypoblast and the epiblast. (3) The ventral layer is termed the *endoderm.* It is thought to consist of cells which originate in the epiblast and migrate inward to displace the cells of the hypoblast.

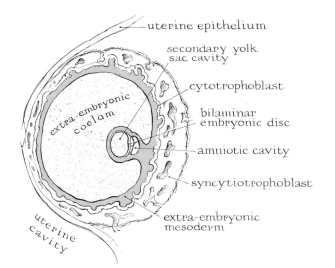

Stage 6 13–15 days (28, 79)
Section of embryonic disc and trophoblast

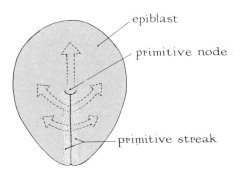

Stage 7 16 days Early 3d week (82)
Dorsal view of the embryonic disc. Arrows indicate the direction of cell migration between the epiblast and the hypoblast.

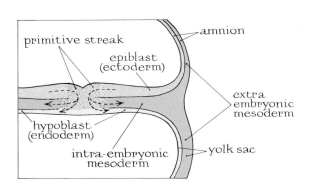

Stage 7 16 days Early 3d week (82)
Transverse section of the embryonic disc through the primitive streak. Arrows indicate the direction of cell migration.

The notochord

As the intra-embryonic mesoderm is being formed, an area of cells termed the *primitive node* appears at the cranial end of the primitive streak. Cells originating in the epiblast invaginate and migrate cranially from the primitive node to form a tubular midline structure termed the *notochordal process.*

Subsequently the notochordal process gives rise to the *notochord,* around which the vertebral bodies and intervertebral disks develop.

The three primary germ layers

The ectoderm, the intra-embryonic mesoderm, and the endoderm are the *three primary germ layers.* Together with the notochordal process they constitute the *trilaminar embryonic disc.* These three primary germ layers are found in all vertebrate embryos, and as a general rule it may be said that in all vertebrates during normal development the ectoderm gives rise to the nervous system and to the epidermis and its derivatives; the endoderm gives rise to the epithelium of the alimentary canal and its derivatives; and the intra-embryonic mesoderm gives rise to most other structures. A more complete list of the derivatives of the germ layers is given in Table 3.

The outline of events as described thus far is consistent with that found in most texts, but for the sake of clarity numerous details and controversial points have been omitted. The reader is referred to Luckett (79), Oppenheimer (81), and O'Rahilly (82) for more complete accounts.

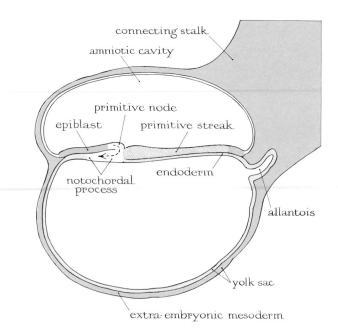

Stage 7 16 days Early 3d week (82)
Sagittal section of the embryonic disc, amnion, and yolk sac. Arrow indicates the direction of cell migration in the formation of the notochordal process.

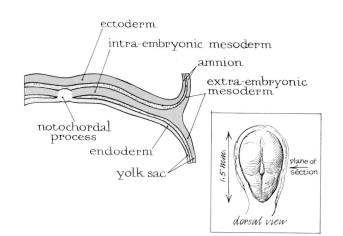

Stage 8 18 days (41)
Transverse section of a pre-somite embryo

Table 2. Origin and Derivation of Tissues in the First Two Weeks (79, 82)

	Zygote	Cleavage-morula	Free blastocyst	Attaching blastocyst	Implantation	Chorionic villi Primitive streak
Days	1	1.5–3	4	5–6	7–12	13
Stages	1	2	3	4	5	6

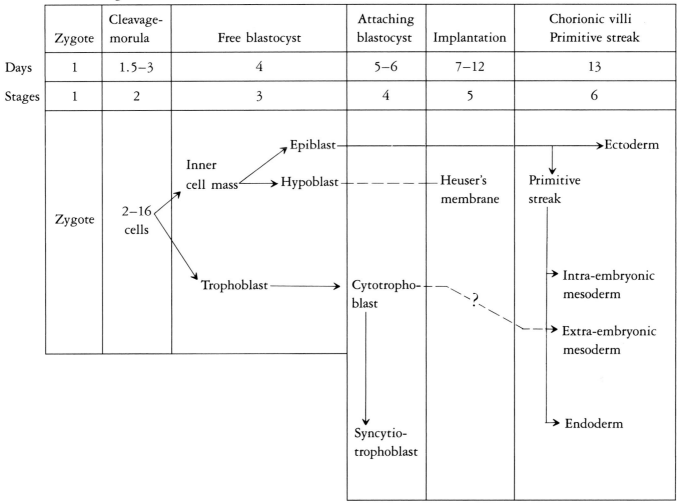

Table 3. The Germ-layer Origin of Human Tissues (1)

Ectoderm	*Mesoderm*	*Endoderm*

1. Epidermis, including:
  cutaneous glands
  hair, nails, lens
2. Epithelium of:
  sense organs
  nasal cavity, sinuses
  mouth, including
    oral glands, enamel
  anal canal
3. Nervous tissue, including:
  hypophysis
  chromaffin tissue
  adrenal medulla
4. Branchial cartilages
5. Muscles of iris
	1. Muscle (all types)
	2. Connective tissue,
	    cartilage, bone, notochord
	3. Blood, bone marrow
	4. Lymphoid tissue
	
	Epithelium of:
	
	5. Blood vessels, lymphatics
	6. Body cavities
	7. Kidney, ureter
	8. Gonads, genital ducts
	9. Suprarenal cortex
	10. Joint cavities, etc.
		Epithelium of:
		
		1. Pharynx, including:
		  root of tongue
		  auditory tube, etc.
		  tonsils, thyroid
		  parathyroids, thymus
		2. Larynx, trachea, lungs
		3. Digestive tube, including
		  parenchyma of associated
		  glands
		4. Bladder
		5. Vagina (all?), vestibule
		6. Urethra, including associated
		  glands

Early differentiation of intra-embryonic mesoderm

During stage 9 three regions can be distinguished within the intra-embryonic mesoderm. They are: (1) the *paraxial mesoderm,* thickened longitudinal bands of tissue which lie on either side of the midline; (2) the *intermediate mesoderm,* a band of tissue lateral to the paraxial mesoderm; and (3) the *lateral plate mesoderm,* a thin sheet of tissue which extends laterally and is continuous with the extra-embryonic mesoderm. (In describing events which occur after the third week, it is customary to refer to the intra-embryonic mesoderm simply as "mesoderm.")

Paraxial mesoderm

Late in the third week (stage 9) the paraxial mesoderm begins to undergo segmentation, forming paired masses termed *somites.* This process continues in a craniocaudal direction throughout the fourth and fifth weeks. Typically there are 4 occipital, 8 cervical, 12 thoracic, 5 lumbar, 5 sacral, and 8 to 10 coccygeal pairs of somites, of which the first occipital and the last 5 or 6 coccygeal somites are resorbed. Not all of these somites are present at one time, however, because the somites which appear first undergo differentiation as the later ones develop.

The early differentiation of the somites

Mesenchyme originating in the ventromedial portion of the somite is termed the *sclerotome.* It surrounds the notochord and forms the vertebral column, the ribs, and the scapula.

The remaining part of the somite is then termed the *dermo-myotome.* Cells originating from the medial aspect of the dermo-myotome proliferate, forming a separate mass of myoblasts (primitive muscle cells) termed the *myotome.* These cells are destined to form most of the skeletal muscles.

After the differentiation of the myotome, the remaining cells are termed the *dermatome.* Cells originating in the dermatome migrate out beneath the ectoderm to form much of the dermis and the subcutaneous tissue.

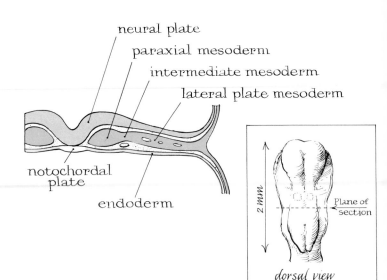

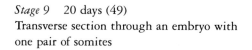

Stage 9 20 days (49)
Transverse section through an embryo with one pair of somites

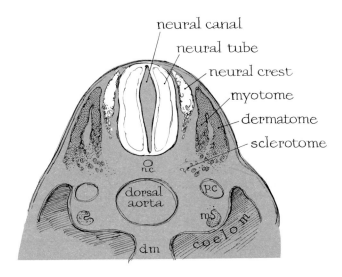

Stage 13 28 days (43, 166, 220)
Transverse section through the spinal cord and adjacent structures

dm: dorsal mesentery
m: mesonephros
nc: notochord
pc: postcardinal vein

Intermediate mesoderm

The intermediate mesoderm opposite the first six somites forms vaguely defined vesicles and nodules which degenerate by the beginning of the fifth week without giving rise to any adult structure (see Torrey [117]). They are of interest, however, because they are homologous with the *pronephros,* a primitive kidney found in certain lower vertebrates. The intermediate mesoderm caudal to the sixth somite forms a solid, unsegmented band of tissue termed the *nephrogenic cord* which gives rise to most of the excretory system.

Lateral plate mesoderm

Early in the fourth week numerous vacuoles appear within the lateral plate mesoderm. These vacuoles rapidly fuse with each other to form the *intra-embryonic coelom,* which will become the pericardial, pleural, and peritoneal cavities. The intra-embryonic coelom divides the lateral plate mesoderm into two layers: *somatic mesoderm* and *splanchnic mesoderm.* Somatic mesoderm is in contact with the ectoderm. It contributes to the body wall, the limb buds, and the muscles of the diaphragm. It also forms the serous membranes which line the body cavities. Splanchnic mesoderm is in contact with the endoderm. It develops into cardiac muscle, the smooth musculature of the viscera, the mesenteries, and the serous membranes which cover the viscera.

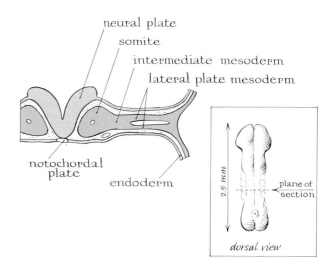

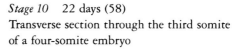

Stage 10   22 days (58)
Transverse section through the third somite of a four-somite embryo

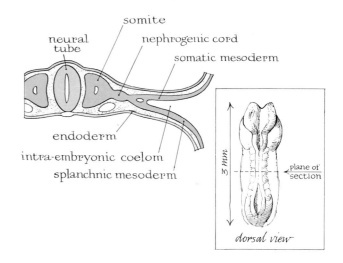

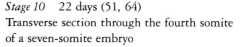

Stage 10   22 days (51, 64)
Transverse section through the fourth somite of a seven-somite embryo

Table 4. The Fate of the Mesoderm (1, 5, 11)

Mesoderm						
	Paraxial mesoderm	Somites	Dermatome	Contributes to dermis (and to skeletal muscles?)		
			Sclerotome	Vertebral column, ribs, scapula		
			Myotome	Pro-otic	Eye muscles	
				Occipital	Tongue muscles	
				Spinal	Epaxial	Extensors of spine
					Hypaxial	Muscles of neck, trunk, and perineum contribute to limb bud and to diaphragm
	Intermediate mesoderm	Pronephros Mesonephros Metanephros		Smooth musculature of urogenital ducts		
	Lateral plate mesoderm	Branchial arch mesoderm	Muscles of mastication, facial expression, phraynx, larynx, etc.			
		Somatic mesoderm	Contributes to limb bud and to diaphragm muscles and to urogenital sphincters, parietal layer of serous membranes			
		Splanchnic mesoderm	Cardiac muscle Most smooth muscle		Visceral part of serous membranes	

The neural plate and the neural tube

During the third week a band of thickened ectoderm termed the *neural plate* appears dorsal to the notochordal plate and adjacent paraxial mesoderm. Shortly thereafter, paired elevations termed *neural folds* develop on either side of the midline. Between the neural folds is a depression termed the *neural groove.* As the neural folds become more prominent, the neural groove deepens, and about the beginning of the fourth week the neural folds meet and fuse dorsally in the region of the fourth pair of somites.

The area of fusion progresses rapidly toward the head and toward the tail, and by the middle of the fourth week the closure of the neural tube is complete except for openings at either end termed the rostral and caudal *neuropores.* The rostral neuropore closes in embryos of about 20 pairs of somites, and the caudal neuropore closes in embryos of about 25 pairs of somites. Closure of the neuropores completes the formation of the neural tube, which constitutes the primordium of the brain and spinal cord (see Figs. 85–88, pp. 120–23).

The neural crest

As the neural tube closes, specialized cells termed *neural crest cells* migrate from the apex of each neural fold. Certain neural crest cells become segmentally arranged on either side of the midline dorsolateral to the neural tube where they give rise to the dorsal root ganglia of the spinal nerves. Other neural crest cells contribute to the formation of the sensory ganglia of cranial nerves V, VII, IX, and X, to the peripheral cells of the autonomic nervous system, and to a variety of other structures.

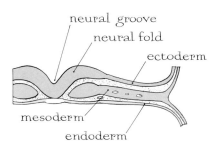

Stage 9 20 days (49)
Transverse section through an embryo having one pair of somites

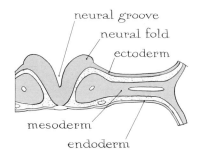

Stage 10 22 days (58)
Transverse section through the third somite of a four-somite embryo

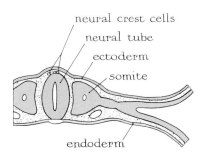

Stage 10 22 days (58)
Transverse section through the fourth somite of a seven-somite embryo

Endoderm

At the end of the third week the endoderm constitutes the inferior layer of the trilaminar embryonic disc and extends peripherally to form the inner layer of the yolk sac. During the fourth week the embryo undergoes a complex series of changes characterized by longitudinal and transverse folding. As a result of these changes the cranial and caudal portions of the endoderm become closed ventrally and are incorporated into the embryonic body, where they form the epithelial lining of the foregut and the hindgut, respectively. (See p. 34.) The part of the endoderm between the foregut and the hindgut is termed the midgut. Ventrally it communicates with the yolk sac via the tubular yolk stalk (see Fig. 12, p. 39).

During further development the endoderm forms the epithelial lining of the digestive tract and its derivatives, including the respiratory system. In addition, it forms the parenchyma of those glands that arise as outgrowths of the digestive system.

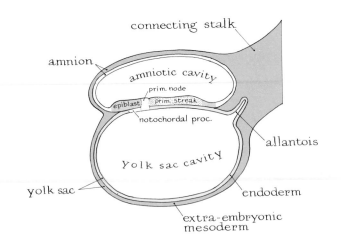

Stage 7 16 days (82)
Sagittal section of the embryo, amnion, and yolk sac of a pre-somite embryo

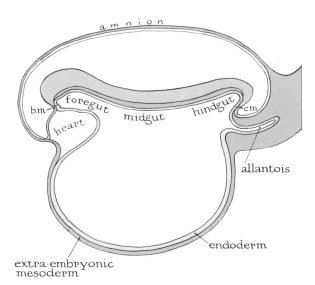

Stage 10 22 days (51) A seven-somite embryo. The endoderm is cut in the sagittal plane slightly to one side of the midline; the rest of the embryo is illustrated schematically in outline.

bm: buccopharyngeal membrane
cm: cloacal membrane

THE DEVELOPMENT OF THE TROPHOBLAST

Syncytiotrophoblast and cytotrophoblast

During and after implantation two types of tissue differentiate within the trophoblast. (1) The *syncytiotrophoblast*: this is the outer multinucleated layer which is actively engaged in the invasion of the endometrium. (2) The *cytotrophoblast*: this portion of the trophoblast consists of individual cells which surround the blastocoele.

Trophoblastic lacunae and intervillous spaces

Early in the second week minute spaces develop within the syncytiotrophoblast. These spaces rapidly become larger and fuse to form a series of confluent channels termed *trophoblastic lacunae*. As the syncytiotrophoblast continues to invade the endometrium it comes into contact with and erodes the walls of the maternal capillaries with the result that maternal blood enters the trophoblastic lacunae. After the development of the chorionic villi the trophoblastic lacunae become the *intervillous spaces*.

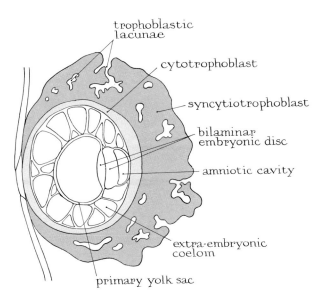

trophoblastic lacunae
cytotrophoblast
syncytiotrophoblast
bilaminar embryonic disc
amniotic cavity
extra-embryonic coelom
primary yolk sac

Stage 5 11–12 days (36, 39)
Section of the blastocyst embedded in the endometrium. For the sake of simplicity individual cells are not illustrated (see Fig. 2).

13

Formation of the chorionic villi

As the result of the formation of the trophoblastic lacunae, the syncytiotrophoblast assumes the form of an irregular network of anastomosing trabeculae. Toward the end of the second week cells originating in the cytotrophoblast invade these trabeculae. The result of this invasion is the formation of numerous cellular columns termed *primary villi.* Each primary villus consists of a core of cells derived from the cytotrophoblast, surrounded by a covering of cells derived from the syncytiotrophoblast (see Fig. 3, p. 19).

During the third week cells originating in the extra-embryonic mesoderm penetrate the primary villi. The resulting structure is termed a *secondary villus,* and consists of an inner core derived from extra-embryonic mesoderm, a middle layer derived from the cytotrophoblast, and an outer covering derived from the syncytiotrophoblast. As the secondary villus develops, cytotrophoblastic cell columns from adjacent villi grow distally and join each other to form a continuous layer termed the *cytotrophoblastic shell* which anchors the villi to the endometrium.

During the latter part of the third week capillaries develop within the mesodermal core of the villus, which is then termed a *tertiary villus.* The capillaries within the villus grow rapidly and soon form anastomoses with branches of the umbilical artery and vein (see Figs. 4 and 5, pp. 20 and 21).

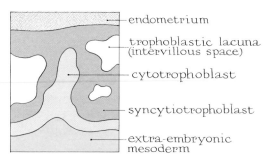

Primary villus

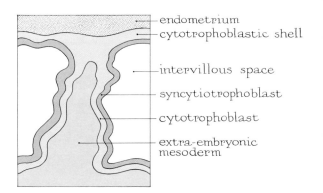

Secondary villus

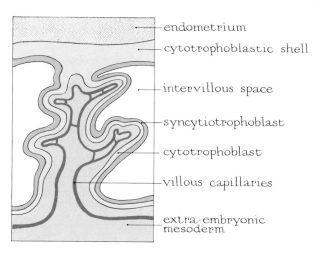

Tertiary villus

Three stages in the development of a chronic villus as seen in schematic longitudinal sections (76, 82)

The chorion

The membrane formed by the extra-embryonic mesoderm and the trophoblast is termed the *chorion*. During the early stages of their development the villi are distributed evenly around the surface of the chorion. During the second and third months, however, the villi near the attachment of the umbilical cord become larger and more abundant, and this area is then termed the *chorion frondosum,* or *bushy chorion*. At the same time, the villi on the rest of the chorion become smaller and finally disappear. This portion of the chorion is then termed the *chorion laeve*, or *smooth part of the chorion*.

The decidua

The mucous membrane of the pregnant uterus is termed the *decidua*. During pregnancy the parts of the decidua are named according to their relationship to the embryo. The part which lines the inner wall of the uterus is the *decidua parietalis*, the part which encloses the embryo is the *decidua capsularis*, and the part which lies between the chorion frondosum and the uterine wall is the *decidua basalis*.

As the embryo increases in size during the second month the double membrane formed by the decidua capsularis and the chorion laeve occupies a larger and larger part of the uterine cavity. During the third and fourth months the decidua capsularis degenerates and the chorion laeve subsequently comes into direct contact with, and fuses with, the decidua parietalis, with the result that the uterine cavity is largely obliterated. Subsequently the amnion, together with its covering of extra-embryonic mesoderm, also makes contact with the chorion, and the chorionic cavity is obliterated.

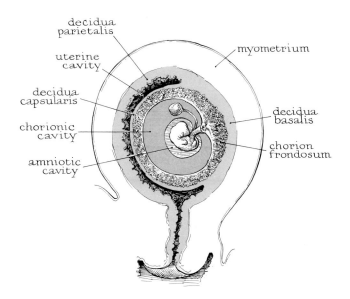

Stage 16 8–11 mm 6th week (11, 76, 78)
Sagittal section of the uterus and fetal membranes

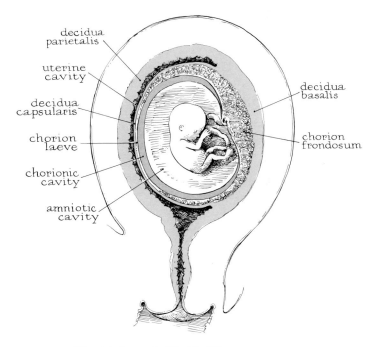

The third month (11, 76, 78)
Sagittal section of the uterus and fetal membranes

THE PLACENTA

The placenta is a composite structure consisting of a fetal part, the chorion frondosum, and a maternal part, the decidua basalis. On the fetal side the villi are attached to the chorionic plate (derived from extra-embryonic mesoderm). On the maternal side they are attached at first to the cytotrophoblastic shell, but during the fourth and fifth months this shell becomes progressively thinner so that during the latter part of the fetal period in many places the villi are attached directly to the decidua basalis.

After delivery the maternal surface of the placenta is seen to consist of ten or more irregular subdivisions termed *lobes*. These lobes are partially separated from each other by pyramidal projections of endometrial tissue termed *decidual septa*. The decidual septa extend from the maternal side of the placenta partway into the intervillous space, but their structure is irregular so that the branches of the villi characteristically extend across the septa and into adjacent lobes. A single lobe may embrace as many as ten or more individual stem villi and their associated branches.

The villi are bathed in maternal blood, which enters the intervillous space via the *spiral arteries* (terminal branches of the arteries which supply the endometrium). The exchange of metabolites between the embryonic blood in the villous capillaries and the maternal blood in the intervillous spaces takes place through the walls of the villi.

This tissue, which is termed the *placental barrier*, changes during the course of pregnancy. Initially it consists of (1) the endothelium of the villous capillary with its basement membrane, (2) the mesodermal tissue of the villus, (3) the cytotrophoblastic layer of the villus with its basement membrane, and (4) the syncytial covering of the villus. During and after the first month, however, the mesodermal and cytotrophoblastic layers become greatly attenuated in the terminal villi so that the placental barrier consists only of the endothelium of the capillary, its basement membrane, and the syncytial covering of the villus.

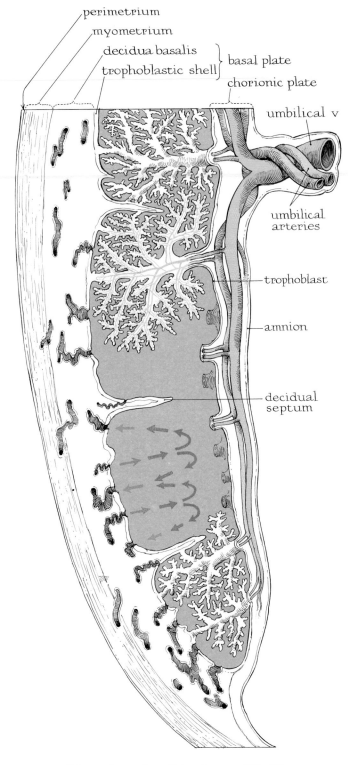

Schematic section of the placenta (76, 83)

16

Illustrated Overview
of the First Two Months

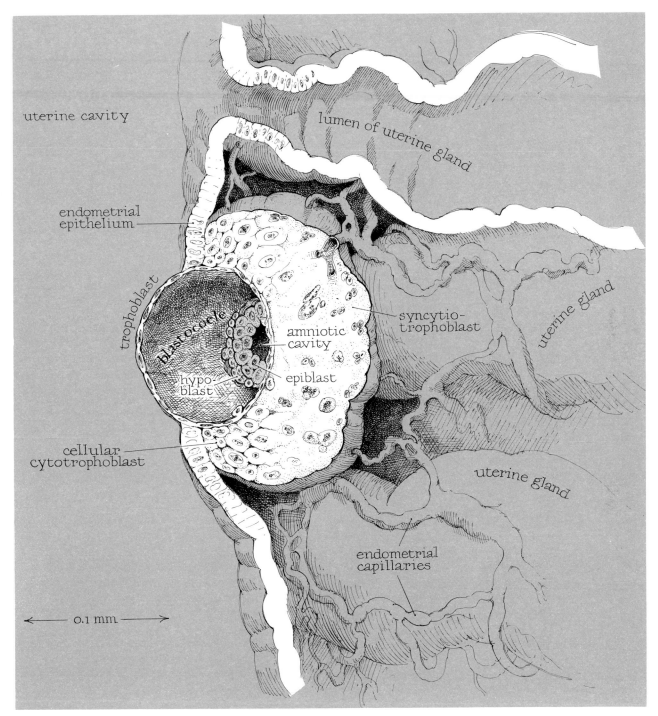

Figure 1. Stage 5a
0.1 mm   7–8 days
(37, 38, 39, 82)
Section of blastocyst
partially implanted in
endometrium

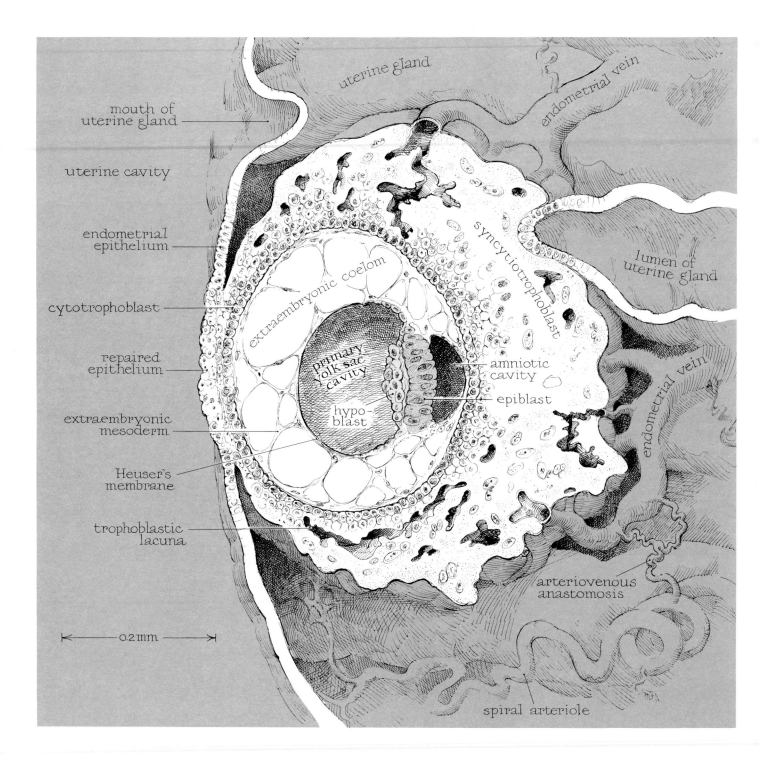

uterine gland

endometrial vein

mouth of
uterine gland

uterine cavity

endometrial
epithelium

cytotrophoblast

repaired
epithelium

extraembryonic
mesoderm

Heuser's
membrane

trophoblastic
lacuna

extraembryonic coelom

syncytiotrophoblast

primary
yolk sac
cavity

hypo-
blast

amniotic
cavity

epiblast

lumen of
uterine gland

endometrial vein

arteriovenous
anastomosis

spiral arteriole

0.2 mm

Figure 2. Stage 5c
0.1–0.2 mm   11–12 days
(36, 39, 42, 82)
Section of blastocyst
completely embedded in
endometrium

18

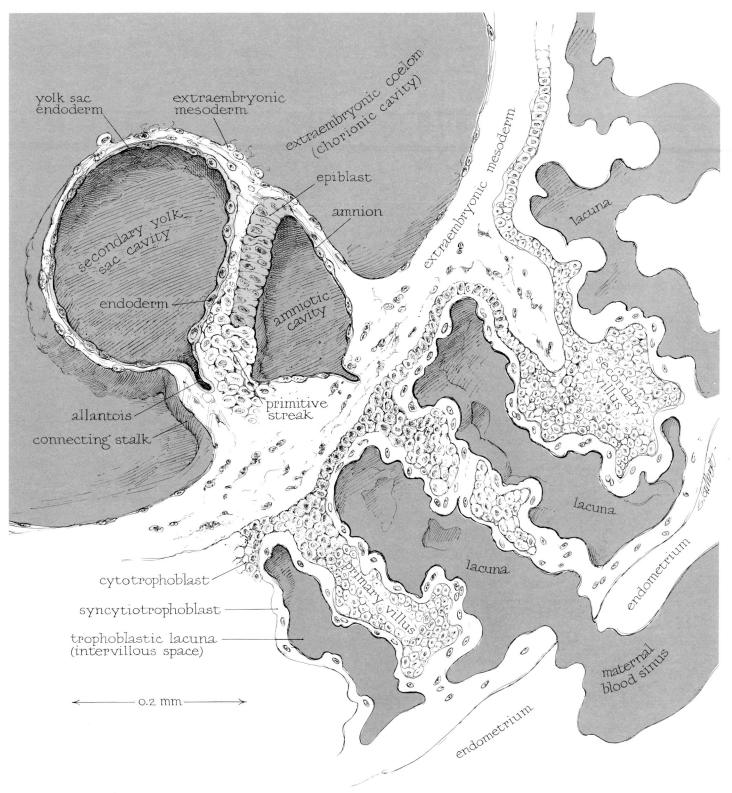

Figure 3. Stage 6
0.2 mm   13–15 days
(28, 42, 59, 71, 82)
Sagittal section of embryo and
related part of chorion

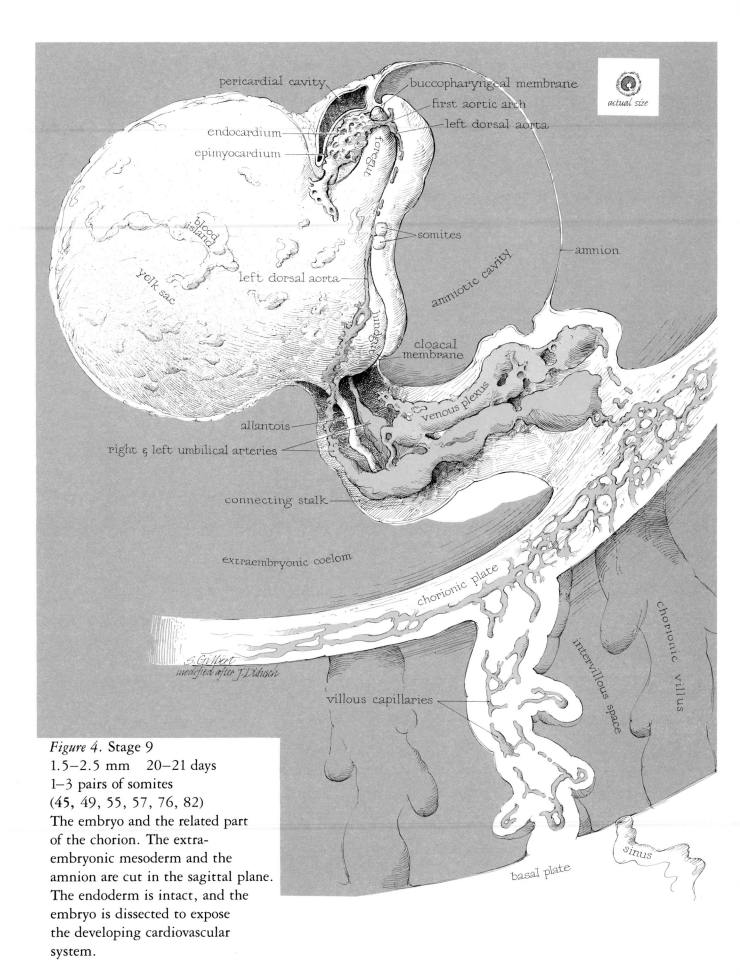

Figure 4. Stage 9
1.5–2.5 mm 20–21 days
1–3 pairs of somites
(**45,** 49, 55, 57, 76, 82)
The embryo and the related part
of the chorion. The extra-
embryonic mesoderm and the
amnion are cut in the sagittal
plane. The endoderm is intact, and the
embryo is dissected to expose
the developing cardiovascular
system.

20

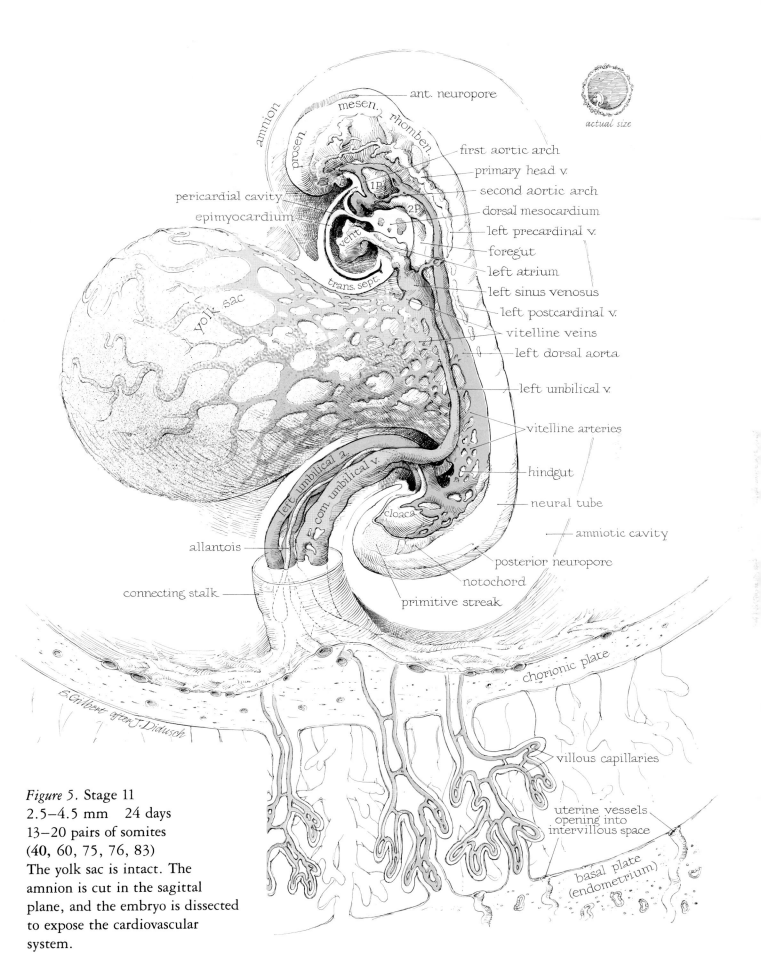

ant. neuropore

actual size

mesen. rhomben.

prosen.

amnion

first aortic arch

primary head v.

second aortic arch

dorsal mesocardium

left precardinal v.

foregut

left atrium

left sinus venosus

left postcardinal v.

vitelline veins

left dorsal aorta

left umbilical v.

vitelline arteries

hindgut

neural tube

amniotic cavity

posterior neuropore

notochord

primitive streak

pericardial cavity

epimyocardium

1D

2P

vent.

trans. sept.

yolk sac

left umbilical a.

con. umbilical v.

cloaca

allantois

connecting stalk

chorionic plate

villous capillaries

uterine vessels opening into intervillous space

basal plate (endometrium)

S. Gilbert after J. Didusch

Figure 5. Stage 11
2.5–4.5 mm   24 days
13–20 pairs of somites
(**40**, 60, 75, 76, 83)
The yolk sac is intact. The
amnion is cut in the sagittal
plane, and the embryo is dissected
to expose the cardiovascular
system.

21

Figure 6. Stage 13
4–6 mm   28 days   30 + pairs of somites
(61, 115, 141, 143, 154, 156)
Superficial dissection. The myotomes and
the lateral body wall have been dissected
to expose underlying structures.

A: allantois
C-1: first cervical neural crest
CC: common cardinal vein
EC: extraembryonic coelom
G: gallbladder
L-1: first lumbar neural crest
L: lung
LA: left atrium
LU: left umbilical vein
LV: left vitelline vein
myo.: myocardium

OV: otic vesicle
P: dorsal pancreatic bud
PC: pericardial cavity
p1, p2, p3, p4: pharyngeal pouches
R: right umbilical artery
RA: right atrium
RU: right umbilical vein
RV: right vitelline vein
S: stomach
T-1: first thoracic neural crest
trig. gang.: trigeminal ganglion
VA: vitelline artery
V: trigeminal nerve
VII: facial nerve
VIII: vestibulocochlear nerve
IX: glossopharyngeal nerve
X: vagus nerve
1-2-3: aortic arches

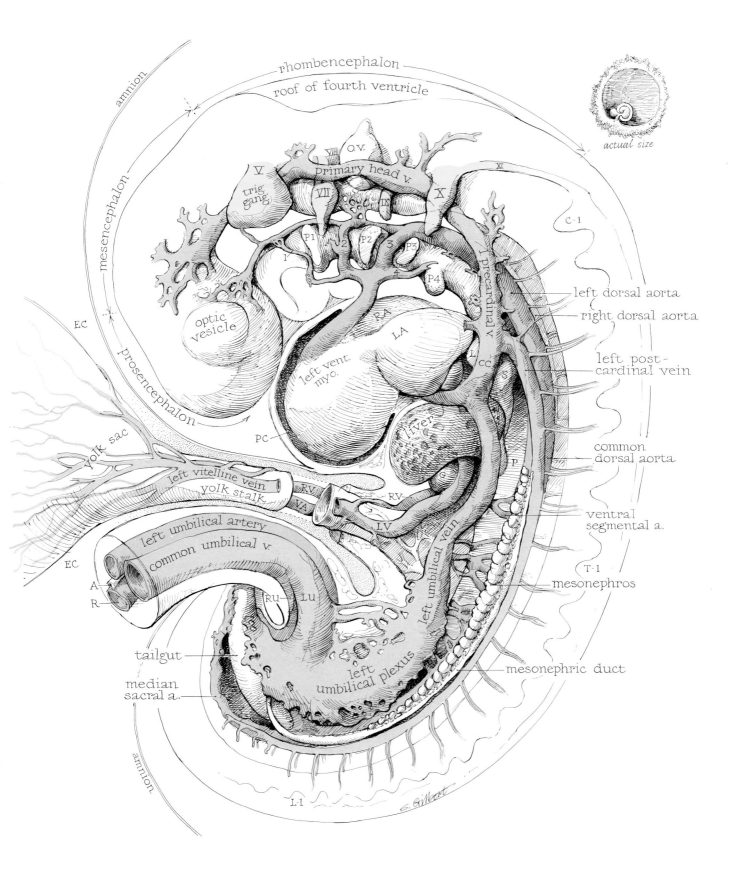

rhombencephalon

roof of fourth ventricle

amnion

mesencephalon

actual size

V
trig. gang.

VI   O.V.
VIII

primary head v.

VII

IX   X

XI

C-1

P1

P2

P3

1

4

P4

I precardinal v.

left dorsal aorta

right dorsal aorta

RA

LA

left post-cardinal vein

EC

prosencephalon

optic vesicle

left vent. myo.

LCC

liver

common dorsal aorta

P

yolk sac

left vitelline vein

yolk stalk

PC

RV

RV

ventral segmental a.

VA

LV

mesonephros

EC

left umbilical artery

common umbilical v.

left umbilical vein

A

Ru   Lu

R

T-1

tailgut

left umbilical plexus

mesonephric duct

median sacral a.

amnion

L-1

S. Gilbert

23

Figure 7. Stage 13
4–6 mm   28 days   30 + pairs of somites
(61, 97, 115, 141, 143)
Deep dissection. The veins, the liver, and
the mesonephroi and their ducts have been
removed to expose the arteries and the alimentary canal. The epimyocardium has been
dissected to expose the interior of the heart.

C-1: first cervical neural crest
endo.: endothelium
H: hepatic diverticulum
L-1: first lumbar neural crest
OV: otic vesicle

P1, P2, P3, P4: pharyngeal pouches
RA: endothelium of right atrium
SV: sinus venosus
T-1: first thoracic neural crest
t sep: transverse septum
trunc. art.: truncus arteriosus
V: trigeminal nerve
VII: facial nerve
VIII: vestibulocochlear nerve
IX: glossopharyngeal nerve
X: vagus nerve
XI: accessory nerve
1-2-3: aortic arches

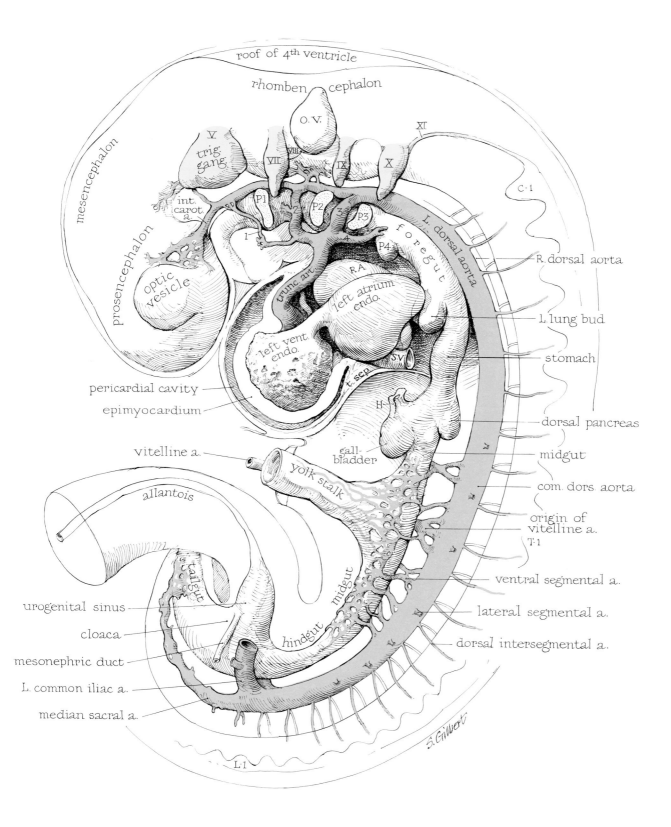

roof of 4ᵗʰ ventricle

rhomben cephalon

O. V.

XI

mesencephalon

V
trig.
gang.

VII

VIII

IX

X

C·1

int.
carot.
a.

P1

P2

P3

L. dorsal aorta

foregut

R. dorsal aorta

prosencephalon

optic
vesicle

trunc. art.

RA

left atrium
endo.

P4

l. lung bud

stomach

left vent.
endo.

SV

t. sep.

H

pericardial cavity

epimyocardium

dorsal pancreas

vitelline a.

gall-
bladder

midgut

yolk stalk

com. dors. aorta

allantois

origin of
vitelline a.

T·1

tailgut

midgut

ventral segmental a.

urogenital sinus

lateral segmental a.

cloaca

hindgut

dorsal intersegmental a.

mesonephric duct

L. common iliac a.

median sacral a.

S. Gilbert

L·1

25

Figure 8. Stage 16
8–11 mm   37 days
(62, 97, 115, 141, 143, 153, 154)
Superficial dissection. Portions of the head
mesenchyme and the lateral body wall have been
removed to expose underlying structures.

A: allantois
C-1: spinal ganglion of first cervical nerve
C: celiac artery
CC: left common cardinal vein
CM: cloacal membrane
DV: ductus venosus
IM: inferior mesenteric artery
L: lens
LU: left umbilical artery
OC: optic cup

OV: otic vesicle
P: portal vein
RU: right umbilical artery
SAP: stem of anterior cerebral plexus
SM: superior mesenteric artery
SMP: stem of middle cerebral plexus
SP: stem of posterior cerebral plexus
TA: truncus arteriosus
trig. gang.: trigeminal ganglion
III: oculomotor nerve
IV: trochlear nerve
V: trigeminal nerve
VII: facial nerve
VIII: vestibulocochlear nerve
IX: glossopharyngeal nerve
X: vagus nerve
XII: hypoglossal nerve

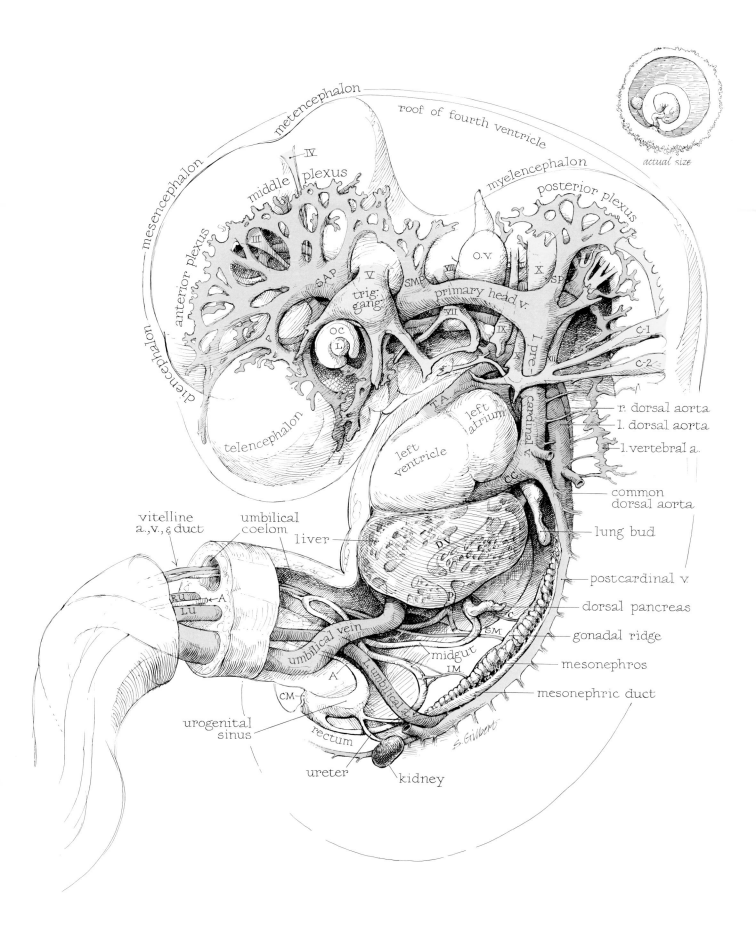

actual size

mesencephalon

metencephalon

roof of fourth ventricle

myelencephalon

posterior plexus

IV

middle plexus

anterior plexus

diencephalon

III

SAP

V

trig. gang.

SMP

OC L.

telencephalon

O.V.

VIII

VII

primary head v.

IX

X

XII

SP

l. pre-cardinal v.

C-1

C-2

r. dorsal aorta

l. dorsal aorta

l. vertebral a.

T.A.

left atrium

left ventricle

CC

common dorsal aorta

lung bud

vitelline a.,v.,& duct

umbilical coelom

liver

DV

RU

LU

A

P

postcardinal v.

dorsal pancreas

C

SM

gonadal ridge

mesonephros

umbilical vein

midgut

IM

mesonephric duct

A

l. umbilical a.

CM

urogenital sinus

rectum

ureter

kidney

S. Gilbert

Figure 9. Stage 16
8–11 mm   37 days
(62, 97, 141, 143)
Deep dissection. The body wall and the
umbilical cord have been cut in the mid-
sagittal plane. The veins, the liver, and
the left mesonephros and its duct have been
removed to expose the arteries and the
alimentary canal. The heart has been cut
to the left of midline in the sagittal plane.

B2: second branchial arch
C-1: spinal ganglion of first cervical nerve
dors. panc.: dorsal pancreas
F-1: foramen primum
F-2: foramen secundum
HV: right hepatocardiac vein
I: interventricular foramen
L: lens
LA: left atrium
LV: left ventricle
MB: mandibular process
MX: maxillary process
OC: optic cup
P-1: first pharyngeal pouch
P-2: second pharyngeal pouch
P-3: third pharyngeal pouch

P-4: fourth pharyngeal pouch
PCA: posterior communicating artery
PT: pulmonary trunk
RD: right dorsal aorta
RU: right umbilical vein
S: sinus venosus
sept. trans.: septum transversum
TA: truncus arteriosus
trig. gang.: trigeminal ganglion
US: urogenital sinus
VP: ventral pancreas
III: oculomotor nerve
IV: trochlear nerve
V: trigeminal nerve
V-1: ophthalmic nerve
V-2: maxillary nerve
V-3: mandibular nerve
VII: facial nerve
VIII: vestibulocochlear nerve
IX: glossopharyngeal nerve
X: vagus nerve
XI: accessory nerve
XII: hypoglossal nerve
3: third aortic arch
4: fourth aortic arch
6: sixth aortic arch

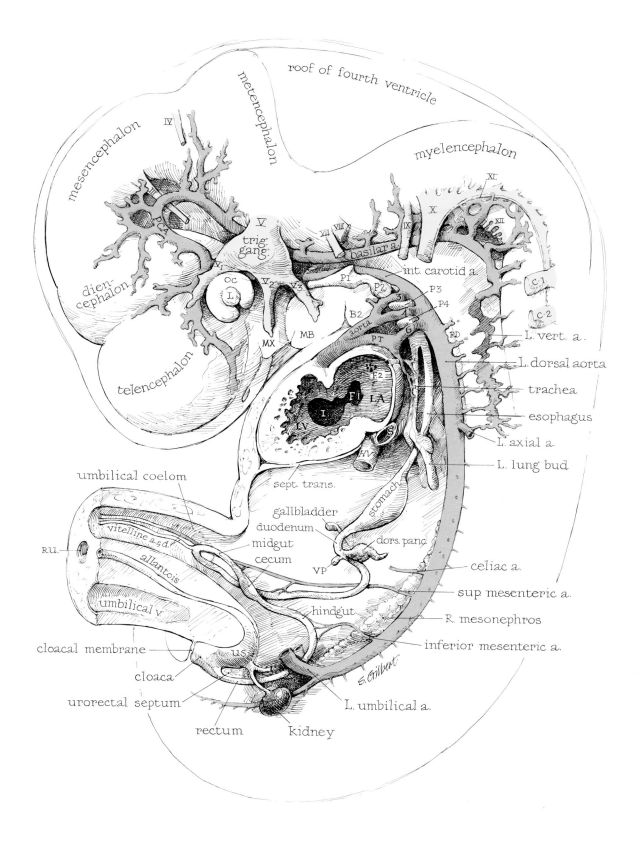

roof of fourth ventricle

mesencephalon

metencephalon

myelencephalon

IV

XI

III

X

V

XII

PCA

trig. gang.

VII VIII

IX

int. carotid a.

C-1

dien-cephalon

V₁

OC

basilar a.

L

V₂

V₃

P1

P2

P3

C-2

telencephalon

MX

MB

B2

aorta

P4

L. vert. a.

PT

4

RD

L. dorsal aorta

F2

trachea

F

LA

esophagus

LV

I

S

L. axial a.

HV

L. lung bud

umbilical coelom

sept. trans.

stomach

vitelline a.g.d.

gallbladder

duodenum

dors. panc.

RU.

midgut

cecum

VP

celiac a.

allantois

sup. mesenteric a.

umbilical v.

hindgut

R. mesonephros

cloacal membrane

inferior mesenteric a.

us.

cloaca

S. Gilbert

urorectal septum

L. umbilical a.

rectum

kidney

Figure 10. Stage 19
16–18 mm   48 days
(63, 97, 115, 141, 143, 149, 154)
Superficial dissection. Portions of the head
mesenchyme and the lateral body wall have
been removed to expose underlying structures.

A: appendix
AA: ascending aorta
BCA: branchiocephalic artery
C-1: spinal ganglion of first cervical nerve
CCA: common carotid artery
DPV: primary head vein
DV: ductus venosus
ECA: external carotid artery
ICA: internal carotid artery
IVC: inferior vena cava
LPC: left postcardinal vein
PCA: posterior communicating artery
PT: pulmonary trunk
PTS: primitive transverse sinus

PV: portal vein
SADP: stem of anterior cerebral plexus
SMDP: stem of middle cerebral plexus
SMV: superior mesenteric vein
SPDP: stem of posterior cerebral plexus
SS: primitive sigmoid sinus
SV: splenic vein
trig gang: trigeminal ganglion
UR: urorectal septum
I: olfactory nerve
II: optic nerve
IV: trochlear nerve
V-1: ophthalmic nerve
V-2: maxillary nerve
V-3: mandibular nerve
VI: abducent nerve
VII: facial nerve
VIII: vestibulocochlear nerve
IX: glossopharyngeal nerve
X: vagus nerve
XII: hypoglossal nerve

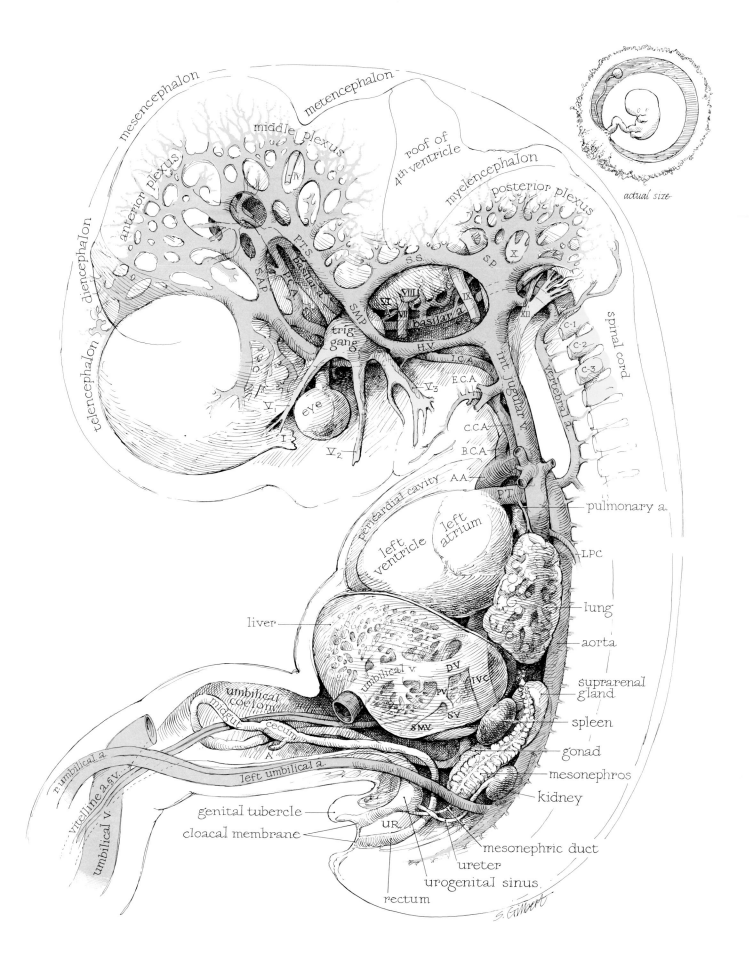

mesencephalon
metencephalon
middle plexus
roof of 4th ventricle
myelencephalon
posterior plexus
actual size
anterior plexus
diencephalon
telencephalon
PT.S.
S.A.P.
basilar a.
I.C.A.
SMP
S.S.
SP
X
VIII
VI
VII
IX
XI
basilar a.
XII
C-1
C-2
C-3
spinal cord
trig. gang.
H.V.
Int. jugular V.
vertebral a.
eye
V₃
I.C.A.
E.C.A.
V
C.C.A.
I
B.C.A.
V₂
A.A.
pericardial cavity
P.T.
pulmonary a.
left atrium
left ventricle
LPC
lung
aorta
liver
DV
IVC
suprarenal gland
umbilical v.
PV
SV
spleen
umbilical coelom
midgut
cecum
SMV
gonad
mesonephros
A
kidney
r. umbilical a.
left umbilical a.
vitelline a. & v.
umbilical v.
genital tubercle
cloacal membrane
UR
mesonephric duct
ureter
urogenital sinus
rectum
S. Gilbert

31

Figure 11. Stage 19
16–18 mm   48 days
(63, 97, 141, 143)
Deep dissection. The body wall and the umbilical cord have been cut in the mid-sagittal plane. The veins, the liver, and the left kidney and mesonephros and their ducts have been removed to expose the arteries and the alimentary canal. The heart has been cut to the left of midline in the sagittal plane.

A: appendix
BCA: brachiocephalic artery
C-1: spinal ganglion of first cervical nerve
CCA: common carotid artery
DA: ductus arteriosus
ECA: external carotid artery
FS: foramen secundum
ICA: internal carotid artery
LA: left atrium
L vent.: left ventricle

N: primitive nasal cavity
OR: primitive oral cavity
P: primitive palate
PT: pulmonary trunk
umb V: umbilical vein
US: urogenital sinus
I: olfactory nerve
II: optic nerve
III: oculomotor nerve
IV: trochlear nerve
V: trigeminal nerve
V-1: ophthalmic nerve
V-2: maxillary nerve
V-3: mandibular nerve
VI: abducent nerve
VII: facial nerve
VIII: vestibulocochlear nerve
IX: glossopharyngeal nerve
X: vagus nerve
XI: accessory nerve
XII: hypoglossal nerve

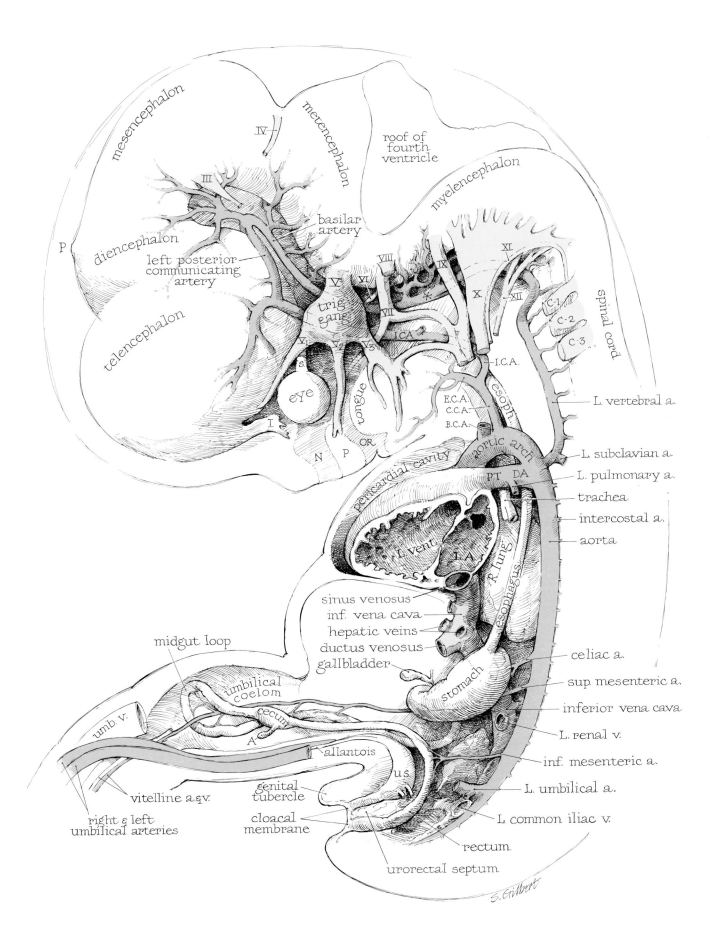

mesencephalon

metencephalon

roof of fourth ventricle

myelencephalon

IV

III

basilar artery

diencephalon

left posterior communicating artery

telencephalon

P

VIII

XI

V VI

trig. gang.

VII

V1 V2 V3

ICA

X

XII

spinal cord

C-1
C-2
C-3

I.C.A.

L. vertebral a.

E.C.A.
C.C.A.
B.C.A.

esoph.

eye

tongue

I

OR.

N P

pericardial cavity

aortic arch

L. subclavian a.

P.T. DA

L. pulmonary a.

trachea

intercostal a.

L. vent

L.A.

R. lung

aorta

esophagus

sinus venosus

inf. vena cava

hepatic veins

ductus venosus

gallbladder

celiac a.

midgut loop

umbilical coelom

cecum

A

stomach

sup. mesenteric a.

inferior vena cava

L. renal v.

umb. v.

allantois

inf. mesenteric a.

genital tubercle

u.s

L. umbilical a.

vitelline a.&v.

cloacal membrane

L. common iliac v.

right & left umbilical arteries

rectum

urorectal septum

S. Gilbert

33

The Digestive and Respiratory Systems

The structure of embryonic gut

The endoderm gives rise to the epithelium lining the alimentary canal, and to the parenchyma of the glands which arise as outgrowths of the primitive gut. The muscles, connective tissues, and peritoneal coverings of the digestive system develop from splanchnic mesoderm.

The digestive system in the fourth week

Early in the fourth week three basic parts of the embryonic digestive system can be distinguished. They are the foregut, the midgut, and the hindgut.

The *foregut* is a blind tube at the cranial end of the body, dorsal to the heart. Its cranial end is closed by the *buccopharyngeal membrane*. The foregut will give rise to the alimentary canal from the mouth to the point where the common bile duct enters the duodenum.

The *midgut* lies between the foregut and the hindgut. Ventrally it communicates with the yolk sac. It will give rise to the alimentary canal from the point where the common bile duct enters the duodenum to a point slightly beyond the middle of the transverse colon.

The *hindgut* is a blind tube at the caudal end of the body. Its dilated terminal portion is termed the *cloaca* and is closed by the *cloacal membrane*. The hindgut gives rise to the alimentary canal from the distal part of the transverse colon to the upper part of the anal canal, and also contributes to the formation of the bladder and the urethra.

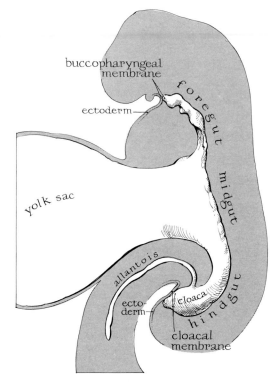

Stage 11 4th week (40)
Left lateral view of gut and yolk sac endoderm

The pharyngeal pouches

During the fourth week four pairs of *pharyngeal pouches* appear as lateral diverticula of the cranial part of the foregut, or primitive pharynx. The pharyngeal pouches contribute to the development of the following structures: first pouch, the middle ear cavity and the auditory tube; second pouch, the palatine tonsil; third pouch, the inferior parathyroid gland and the thymus; fourth pouch, the superior parathyroid gland.

A smaller fifth pharyngeal pouch or *ultimobranchial body* appears to be attached to the fourth pouch. The ultimobranchial bodies are incorporated into the thyroid gland as the parafollicular cells.

The primordium of the thyroid gland originates as a diverticulum from the floor of the pharynx. It migrates caudally, arriving at its final destination ventral to the trachea during the seventh week.

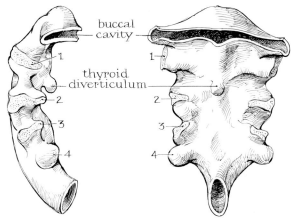

LATERAL VIEW   VENTRAL VIEW

Stage 12   4th week (103)
Lateral and ventral views of the pharyngeal endoderm

The esophagus and the stomach

About the end of the fourth week the stomach makes its appearance as a dilation of the foregut dorsal to the heart. The esophagus develops from the portion of the foregut between the pharynx and the stomach.

During the fifth and sixth week the head, heart, and lungs develop rapidly. At the same time, the esophagus becomes longer and the stomach moves to a more caudal position. By the sixth week the stomach begins to assume its definitive shape. During weeks six and seven it undergoes further descent, growth, and apparent rotation, so that the long dorsal border moves to the left, becoming the greater curvature, and the shorter ventral border moves to the right, becoming the lesser curvature.

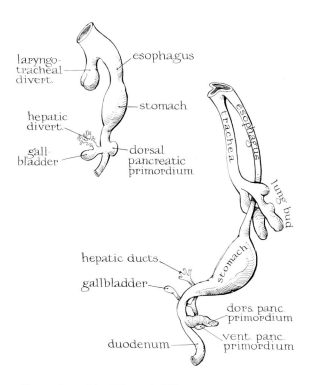

Above: *Stage 14*   5th week (61)
Below: *Stage 16*   6th week (62)
The development of the endodermal components of the esophagus, stomach, and related structures

35

The liver

Early in the fourth week the primordium of the liver (the *hepatic diverticulum*) can be identified as an area of rapidly proliferating endodermal cells which originate from the ventral wall of the gut below the stomach. They invade the *transverse septum* (a sheet of mesoderm between the heart and the yolk stalk) and subsequently give rise to the parenchyma of the liver and to the epithelium of the biliary tract.

Mesenchymal cells in the transverse septum form the sinusoids of the liver, which subsequently unite with invading branches of the vitelline and umbilical veins. Mesenchyme originating in the transverse septum also forms the stroma and the fibrous and serous coverings of the liver as well as the connective tissue and smooth muscle of the biliary tract.

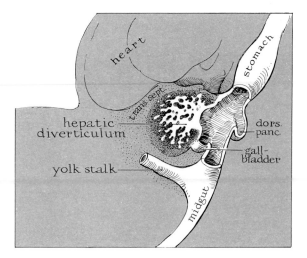

Stage 13 4 weeks (61)
The hepatic diverticulum and the adjacent portion of the gut endoderm are cut in the midsagittal plane.

The pancreas

The pancreas arises from dorsal and ventral primordia. During the fourth week the *dorsal primordium* appears opposite the hepatic diverticulum. The ventral primordium appears during the fifth week. It is usually an outgrowth of the hepatic diverticulum, but it may also arise separately from the duodenum.

The dorsal primordium grows more rapidly than the ventral primordium and soon extends into the dorsal mesentery. During the sixth week the ventral primordium migrates dorsally behind the duodenum to assume a position in the dorsal mesentery. During the seventh week the two primordia unite. The ventral primordium forms the uncinate process and much of the head of the pancreas, while the dorsal primordium forms the body and the tail.

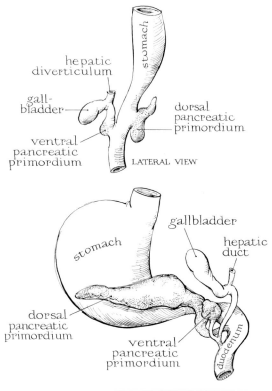

Above: *Stage 15* 5th week (97)
Left lateral view of the pancreatic primordia
Below: *Stage 17* 6th week (97)
Dorsal view of the pancreatic primordia

The midgut

During the fourth week the communication between the midgut and the yolk stalk becomes greatly reduced in size. By the beginning of the fifth week the midgut is a straight tube which is attached to the dorsal body wall by the dorsal mesentery and communicates with the yolk sac via a slender duct termed the *yolk stalk*.

During weeks five and six the midgut increases in length, forming a loop which extends into the *umbilical coelom* (a cavity within the expanded proximal part of the umbilical cord). About the middle of the sixth week the rudiment of the cecum and the appendix can be seen as a dilation in the distal limb of the midgut loop. Toward the end of the sixth week the loop undergoes rotation with the result that the proximal limb comes to lie to the right of and inferior to the distal limb. While in the umbilical coelom the proximal limb undergoes great elongation and coiling and the entire midgut loop undergoes further rotation. During the tenth week the midgut returns to the abdominal cavity.

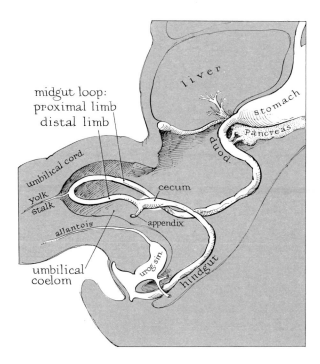

Stage 17   6th week (62)
Left lateral view of the midgut and hindgut. The liver and the body wall are cut in the midsagittal plane.

The hindgut

During weeks five and six the *urorectal septum* (a wedge of mesoderm between the allantois and the hindgut) grows caudally toward the cloacal membrane. As it does so it divides the cloaca into a dorsal part, which will become the rectum and the upper part of the anal canal, and a ventral part termed the *urogenital sinus*. (The further development of the urogenital sinus is described on page 47.) Late in the seventh week the cloacal membrane ruptures, with the result that the anal canal and the urogenital sinus open independently into the amniotic cavity.

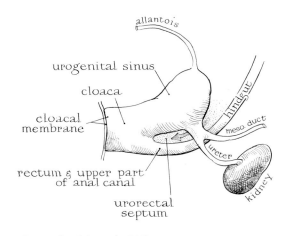

Stage 16   6th week (115)
Left lateral view of the urogenital sinus, cloaca, and hindgut

The larynx, trachea, and lungs

During the fourth week a ventral outgrowth of the foregut endoderm (termed the *laryngo-tracheal diverticulum*) appears just caudal to the pharynx. It will give rise to the lining epithelia and glands of the larynx, the trachea, and the bronchi, and to the epithelium of the alveoli. The smooth muscles, connective tissues, blood vessels, and lymphatics associated with these structures originate from splanchnic mesoderm.

During the fifth and sixth weeks the laryngotracheal diverticulum grows caudally, forming a tube (the primordium of the trachea) which forks to form paired lung buds. By repeated branching the lung buds and their surrounding mesenchyme give rise to the bronchi and the lungs. By the end of the fourth month the principal subdivisions of the bronchi have been established, and between months four and six pulmonary arterioles and capillaries develop rapidly. By the sixth month the lungs are capable of sustaining life in the event of premature birth.

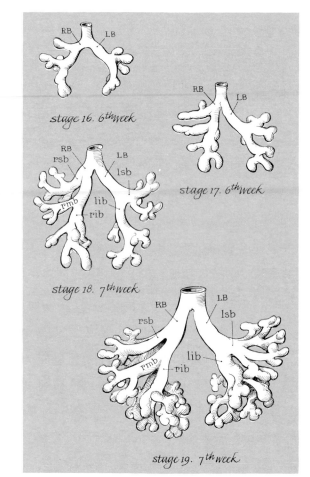

Ventral views of the developing lung buds (104)

RB: right bronchus
rsb: right superior lobe bronchus
rmb: right middle lobe bronchus
rib: right inferior lobe bronchus
LB: left bronchus
lsb: left superior lobe bronchus
lib: left inferior lobe bronchus

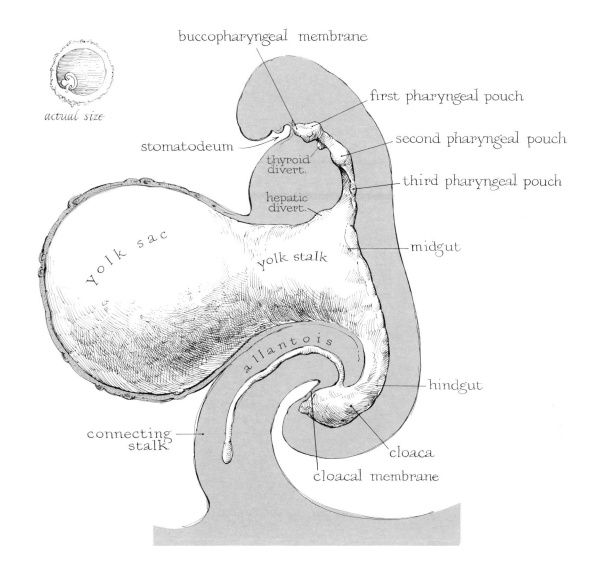

actual size

buccopharyngeal membrane

first pharyngeal pouch

second pharyngeal pouch

third pharyngeal pouch

stomatodeum

thyroid divert.

hepatic divert.

midgut

yolk sac

yolk stalk

allantois

hindgut

connecting stalk

cloaca

cloacal membrane

Figure 12. Stage 11
2.5–4.5 mm   24 days
13–20 pairs of somites
(**40,** 60, 97, 100)
Left lateral view. The endoderm is intact;
the embryo is cut in the mid-sagittal plane
and represented schematically in outline.

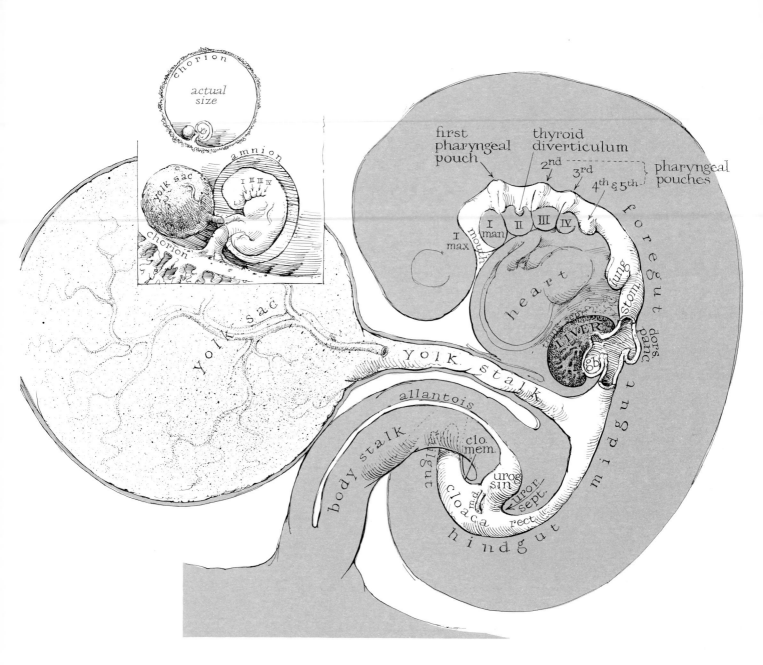

Figure 13. Stage 13
4–6 mm   28 days
30 or more pairs of somites
(**61**, 97, 100)
The liver and adjacent endoderm are cut in the mid-sagittal plane. The rest of the endoderm and its derivatives are intact. The embryo is cut in the mid-sagittal plane and represented schematically in outline.

clo. mem.: cloacal membrane
dors. panc.: dorsal pancreas
gb: gallbladder
md: mesonephric duct
trans. sept.: transverse septum
uror. sept.: urorectal septum
I max.: first branchial arch
  (maxillary process)
I man.: first branchial arch
  (mandibular process)
II: second branchial arch
III: third branchial arch
IV: fourth branchial arch

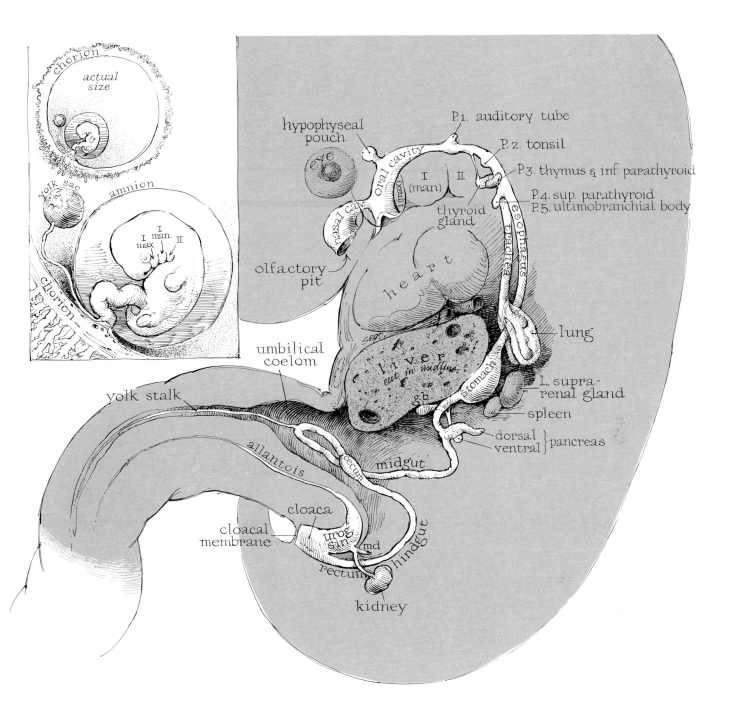

Figure 14. Stage 16
8–11 mm   37 days
(62, 97, 100, 226)
The umbilical cord, ventral body wall, and
liver are cut in the mid-sagittal plane. The
digestive and respiratory systems are intact,
and the rest of the embryo is seen schematically
in outline.

gb: gallbladder
md: mesonephric duct
P1, P2, P3, P4: pharyngeal pouches
sept.: septum transversum
urog. sin.: urogenital sinus
I max.: first branchial arch
   (maxillary process)
I man.: first branchial arch
   (mandibular process)
II: second branchial arch

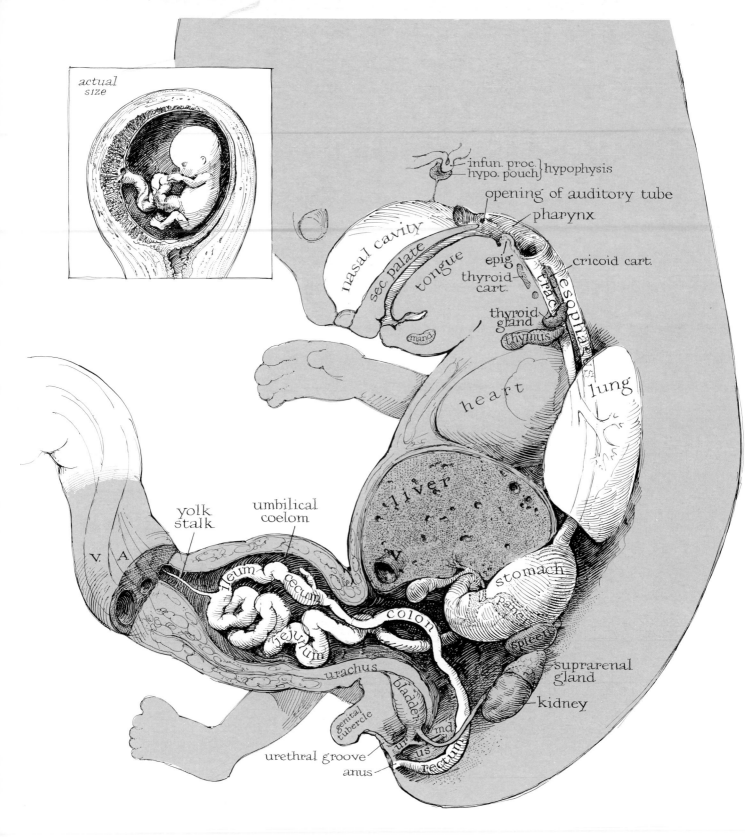

Figure 15. Stage 23
27 mm   57 days
(63, 84, 89, 97, 100, 104)
The umbilical cord, the ventral body wall,
the liver, the mouth and the pharynx are cut
in the mid-sagittal plane. The rest of the
embryo is seen schematically in outline.

A: left umbilical artery
md: mesonephric duct
ur: urethra
us: urorectal septum
V: umbilical vein

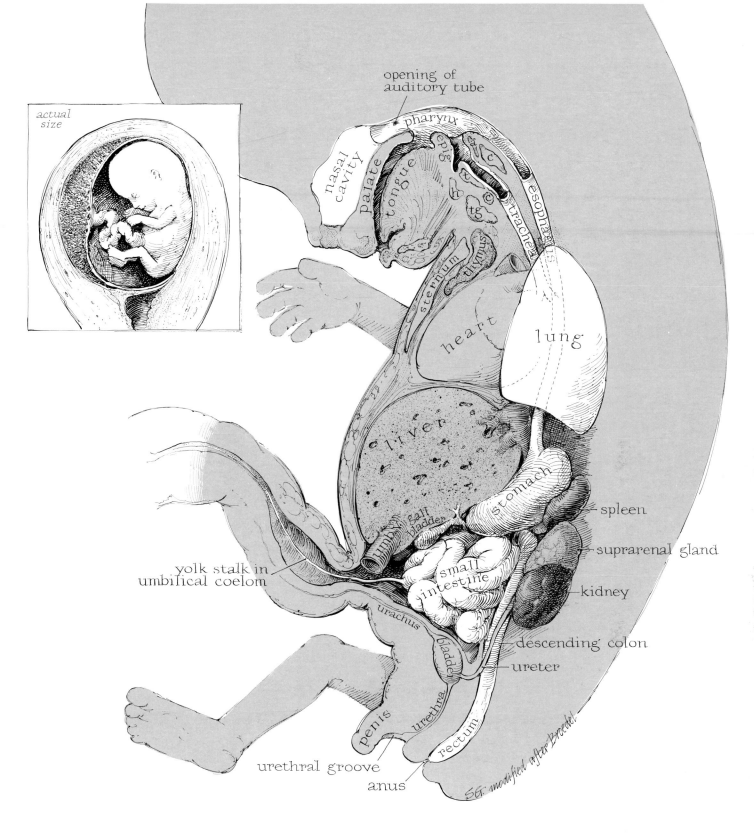

Figure 16. Early fetal period
50 mm   10 weeks
(**85**, 97, 100, 103)
The umbilical cord, the ventral body wall,
the liver, the mouth and the pharynx are cut
in the mid-sagittal plane. The rest of the embryo
is seen schematically in outline.

a: arytenoid cartilage
c: cricoid cartilage
h: hyoid bone
t: thyroid cartilage
tg: thyroid gland

The Urogenital System

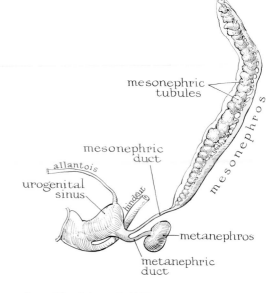

The mesonephros and the male genital tract

During the latter part of the fourth week the nephrogenic cords (see p. 7) give rise to the *mesonephroi*, prominent organs which extend throughout much of the coelomic cavity during the fifth and sixth weeks. Each mesonephros contains forty or more *mesonephric tubules*. These tubules empty into the *mesonephric (Wolffian) duct*, which in turn empties into the cloaca. In fishes, reptiles, and amphibians the mesonephros persists as a major portion of the functional kidney in the adult, but in mammals it degenerates during the latter part of the embryonic period.

In females the mesonephros disappears almost completely, leaving only minute vestiges within the broad ligament. In both males and females the mesonephric duct contributes to the formation of the trigone of the bladder. In males the mesonephric duct plays an important role in the development of the genital tract by contributing to the formation of the epididymis, the ductus deferens, the ejaculatory duct, and the seminal vesicle.

Stage 16   6th week (115)
Lateral view of the left mesonephros, metanephros, and urogenital sinus

The metanephros

The *metanephros*, or permanent adult kidney, begins to develop about the middle of the fifth week. Near the point where the mesonephric duct joins the cloaca an outgrowth of the mesonephric duct termed the *metanephric diverticulum* grows into the caudal part of the nephrogenic cord. The metanephric diverticulum forms the ureter, the pelvis, the calyces, and the collecting ducts of the metanephros. The nephrogenic cord gives rise to the nephrons of the metanephros. The metanephroi originate in the pelvis but gradually migrate cranially, so that by the end of the embryonic period they lie in the upper part of the abdomen.

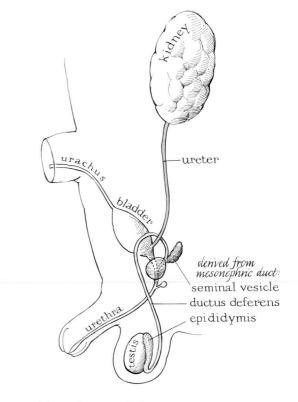

The male urogenital system at term

The female genital tract

The uterus and the uterine tubes develop from the *paramesonephric (Müllerian) ducts* and adjacent mesenchyme. The paramesonephric ducts originate during the sixth week with the invagination of coelomic epithelium into the underlying mesenchyme near the cranial ends of the mesonephric ducts. From this point they grow caudally along the lateral edges of the mesonephric ducts, crossing them ventrally as they approach the urogenital sinus. Toward the end of the eighth week the caudal ends of the paramesonephric ducts meet in the midline dorsal to the urogenital sinus, where they unite to form a fused portion termed the *uterovaginal primordium* which contacts the dorsal wall of the urogenital sinus.

The unfused portions of the paramesonephric ducts give rise to the epithelial lining of the uterine tubes; the uterovaginal primordium gives rise to the epithelial lining of the uterus and most of the vagina. The musculature and peritoneal covering of the female genital tract are derived from adjacent mesenchyme.

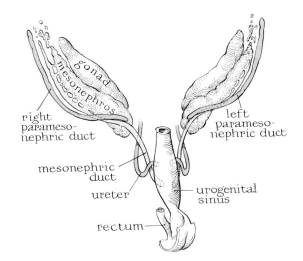

Stage 21 8th week (108)
Ventral view of the paramesonephric ducts and related structures

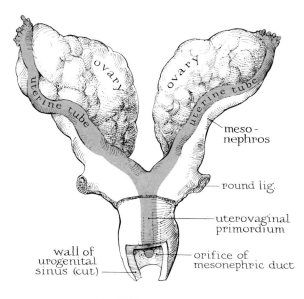

36 mm 9th week (108)
Ventral view of the uterus and ovaries

The gonads

During the fourth week the coelomic epithelium and the underlying mesenchyme medial to the mesonephroi thicken, forming paired *gonadal ridges*. About the same time, primordial germ cells originate in the wall of the yolk sac near the allantois and begin to migrate toward the gonadal ridges. As the ridges grow, solid cord-like extensions of coelomic epithelium termed *primary sex cords* penetrate the underlying mesenchyme. During the sixth week the primordial germ cells reach the gonadal ridges and become embedded within the primary sex cords.

There are no apparent differences in the gonads of male and female embryos until the eighth week when the primary sex cords begin to differentiate. The primary sex cords in the male form the *rete testis* and the seminiferous tubules; those of the female form the *follicular cells* of the *ovarian follicles*.

During the latter part of the embryonic period the testes become rounded and descend from their original position in the abdominal cavity. By the middle of the third month they lie near the internal inguinal ring where they remain until the seventh month, when they pass through the inguinal canal and into the scrotum.

The ovaries, like the testes, become rounded during fetal development. However, they descend only a relatively short distance and take up a position within the pelvic cavity.

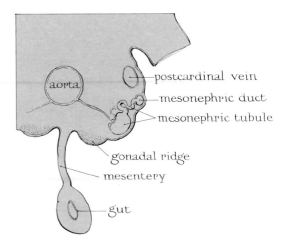

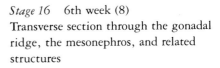

Stage 16   6th week (8)
Transverse section through the gonadal ridge, the mesonephros, and related structures

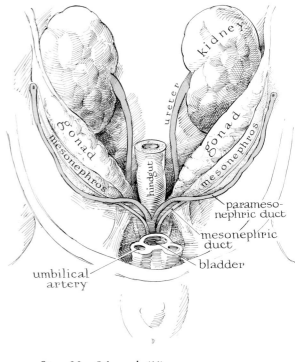

Stage 23   8th week (11)
Ventral view of the gonads and related structures

The urinary bladder and the urethra

In a four-week-old embryo the caudal end of the cloaca is closed by the *cloacal membrane*. Between weeks five and seven a wedge of mesoderm termed the *urorectal septum* grows caudally toward the cloacal membrane, dividing the cloaca into a dorsal part, which will become the rectum and the upper part of the anal canal, and a ventral part, termed the *urogenital sinus*. About the time the partition of the cloaca is completed, the cloacal membrane ruptures, with the result that the anal canal and the urogenital sinus open independently into the amniotic cavity.

The upper part of the urogenital sinus between the allantois and the mesonephric ducts forms the mucosa of the urinary bladder. In the male, the lower part of the urogenital sinus gives rise to all but the most distal portion of the mucosa of the urethra. In the female the mucosa of the urethra is formed by the short portion of the urogenital sinus between the openings of the ureters and the openings of the mesonephric ducts, and the remainder of the urogenital sinus gives rise to the mucosa of the vestibule and probably to part of the vaginal mucosa. In both males and females the muscular portions of the bladder and the urethra are formed from adjacent splanchnic mesoderm during the third month.

During the latter part of the embryonic period the lumen of the allantois becomes occluded by connective tissue, forming a fibrous cord termed the *urachus*. In the adult the urachus persists as the *middle umbilical ligament*, which extends along the midline of the ventral abdominal wall from the bladder to the umbilicus.

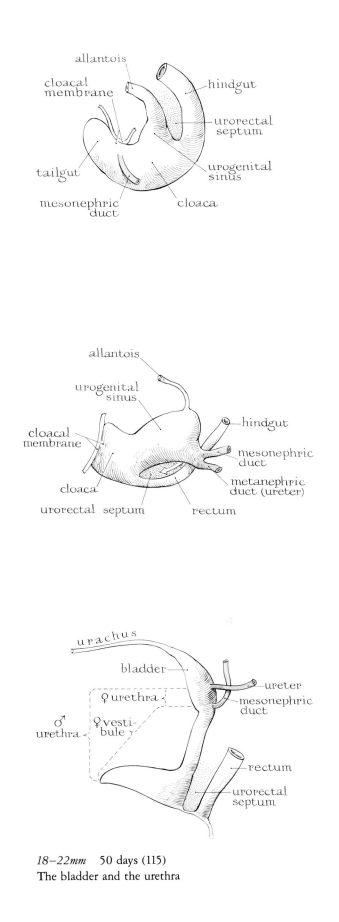

18–22mm 50 days (115)
The bladder and the urethra

The external genitalia

During the sixth week an elevation termed the *genital tubercle* develops anterior to the cloacal membrane. Its caudal surface is marked by a trough-like depression termed the *urethral groove*, into which the lower part of the urogenital sinus opens. On either side of the urethral groove are elevations termed *urogenital folds*, and lateral to the genital tubercle are paired ridges termed *labioscrotal swellings*.

At the end of the embryonic period the external genitalia of the male and the female are similar in appearance, but during the third month the genital tubercle in the male becomes a recognizable penis and the labioscrotal swellings fuse to form the scrotum. Toward the end of the third month the urogenital folds fuse in the midline, transforming the urogenital groove of the male into the *cavernous urethra*. The urethra at this time, however, does not extend to the end of the glans. The distal part of the urethra and the definitive *external urethral orifice* are formed during the fourth month by the ingrowth of ectodermal cells from the tip of the glans.

In the female the genital tubercle becomes the clitoris. The urogenital folds remain unfused and become the labia minora, while the labioscrotal swellings become the labia majora.

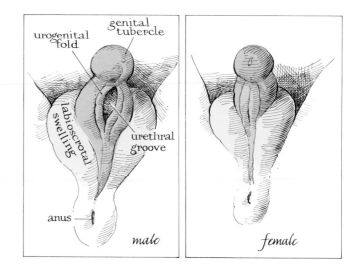

The external genitalia in the ninth week (116)

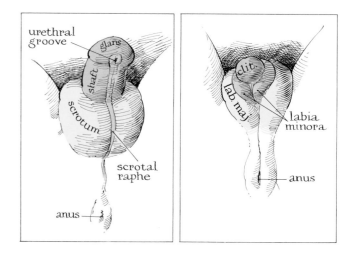

The external genitalia in the tenth week (116)

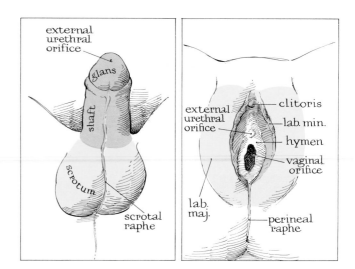

The external genitalia at term

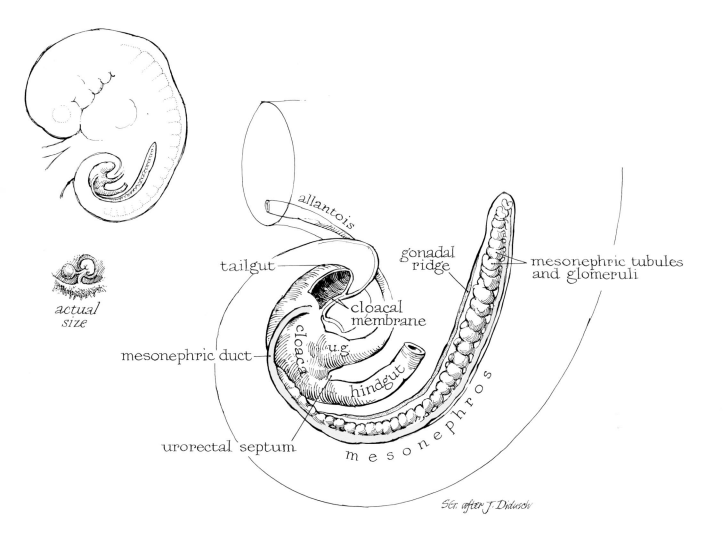

actual
size

allantois

tailgut

cloacal
membrane

gonadal
ridge

mesonephric tubules
and glomeruli

mesonephric duct

cloaca

u.g.

hindgut

urorectal septum

m e s o n e p h r o s

S.G. after J. Didusch

Figure 17. Stage 13
4–6 mm   28 days
30 or more pairs of somites
(98, 109, 113, **115**)
Left lateral view. For the sake of simplicity
the paired structures of the urogenital system
are shown on the left side only. The lateral
wall of the tailgut has been removed to reveal
the cloacal membrane.

ug: urogenital sinus

49

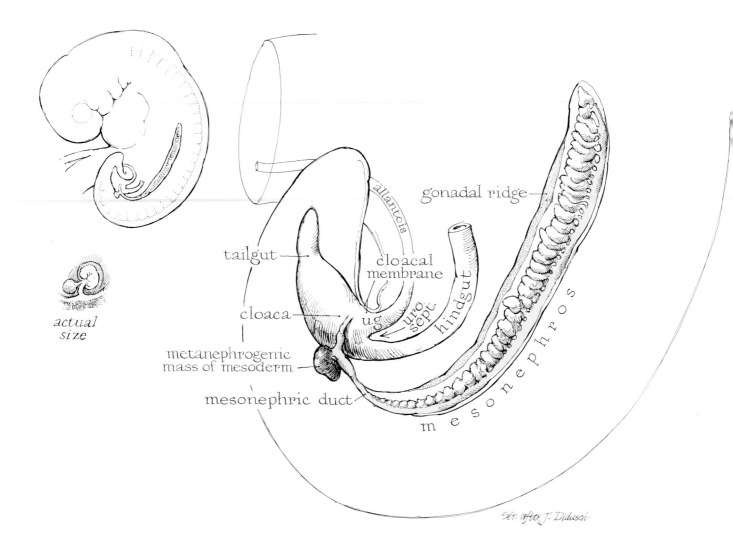

actual
size

gonadal ridge

allantois

tailgut

cloacal
membrane

cloaca

uro.
sept.

hindgut

u.g.

metanephrogenic
mass of mesoderm

mesonephric duct

m e s o n e p h r o s

Sk. after J. Didusch.

Figure 18. Stage 14
5–7 mm   32 days
(61, 98, 105, 109, 113, **115**)

ug: urogenital sinus
uro. sept.: urorectal septum

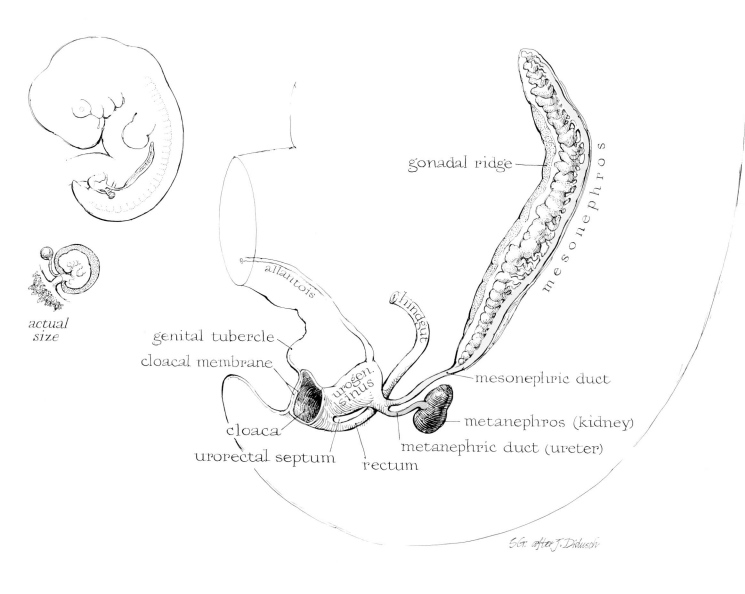

actual
size

gonadal ridge

mesonephros

allantois

hindgut

genital tubercle

cloacal membrane

urogen. sinus

mesonephric duct

metanephros (kidney)

cloaca

urorectal septum

metanephric duct (ureter)

rectum

SG. after J. Didusch

Figure 19. Stage 16
8–11 mm   37 days
(101, 109, 113, 114, **115**)
The left lateral wall of the cloaca has been
removed.

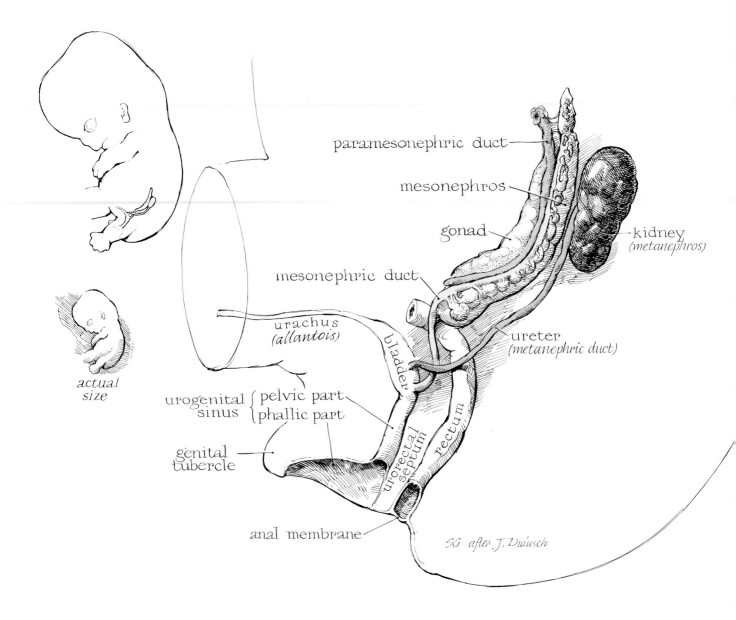

paramesonephric duct

mesonephros

gonad

kidney
(metanephros)

mesonephric duct

urachus
(allantois)

ureter
(metanephric duct)

bladder

urogenital { pelvic part
sinus { phallic part

urorectal septum

rectum

genital
tubercle

anal membrane

SG after J. Drausch

Figure 20. Stage 20
18–22 mm   50 days
(98, 101, 109, 113, **115**)
In this and subsequent illustrations the
left lateral wall of the lower part of the
urogenital sinus has been removed.

actual
size

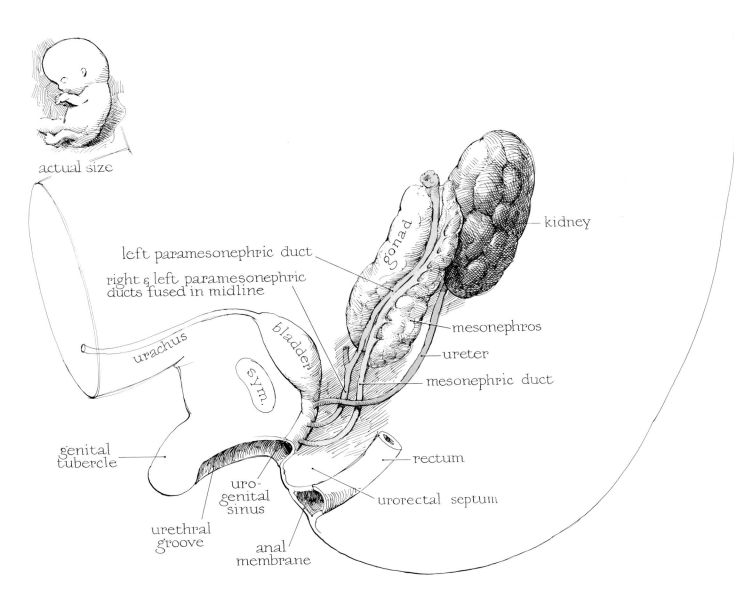

actual size

left paramesonephric duct

right & left paramesonephric
ducts fused in midline

urachus

bladder

sym.

gonad

kidney

mesonephros

ureter

mesonephric duct

genital
tubercle

uro-
genital
sinus

urethral
groove

anal
membrane

rectum

urorectal septum

Figure 21. Stage 23
27–31 mm   57 days
(63, 101, 105, 109, 113, 116)

sym: pubic symphysis

53

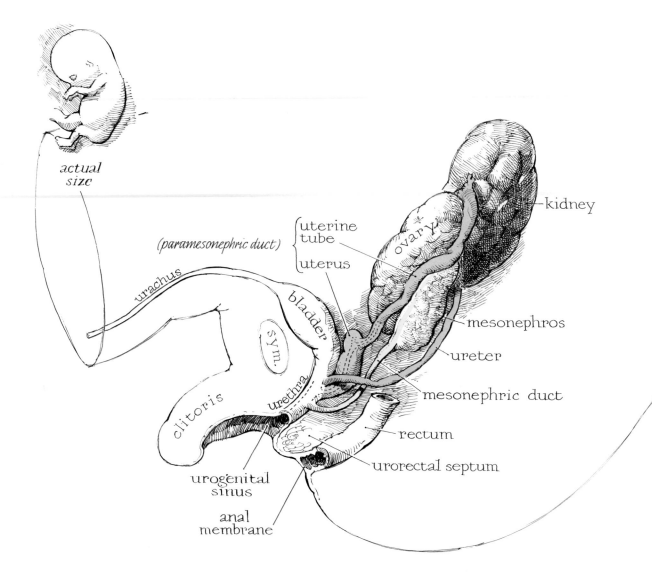

actual
size

(paramesonephric duct)

urachus

uterine
tube

uterus

kidney

ovary

bladder

sym.

mesonephros

ureter

urethra

mesonephric duct

clitoris

rectum

urogenital
sinus

urorectal septum

anal
membrane

Figure 22. Early fetal period
35 mm   8 weeks
(101, 108, 109, 110, 114, 116)
Female urogenital system

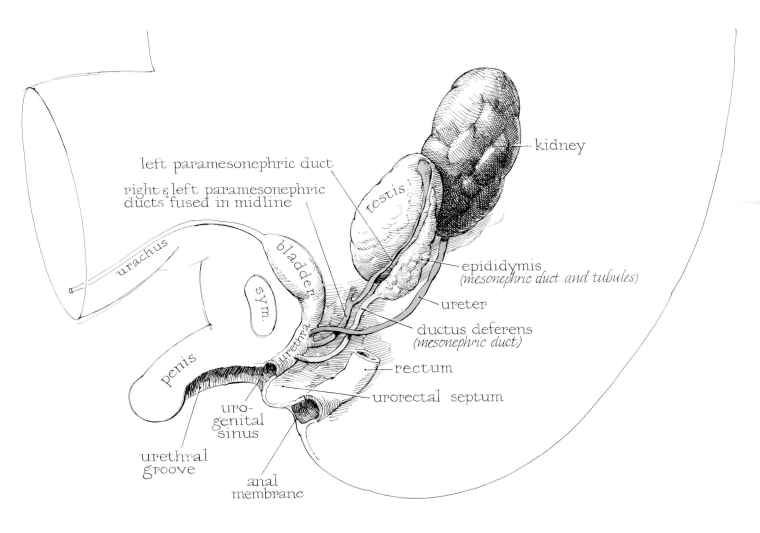

left paramesonephric duct

right & left paramesonephric
ducts fused in midline

urachus

bladder

sym.

penis

urethra

urogenital
sinus

urethral
groove

anal
membrane

kidney

testis

epididymis
(mesonephric duct and tubules)

ureter

ductus deferens
(mesonephric duct)

rectum

urorectal septum

Figure 23. Early fetal period
35 mm   8 weeks
(101, 106, 109, 114, 116)
Male urogenital system

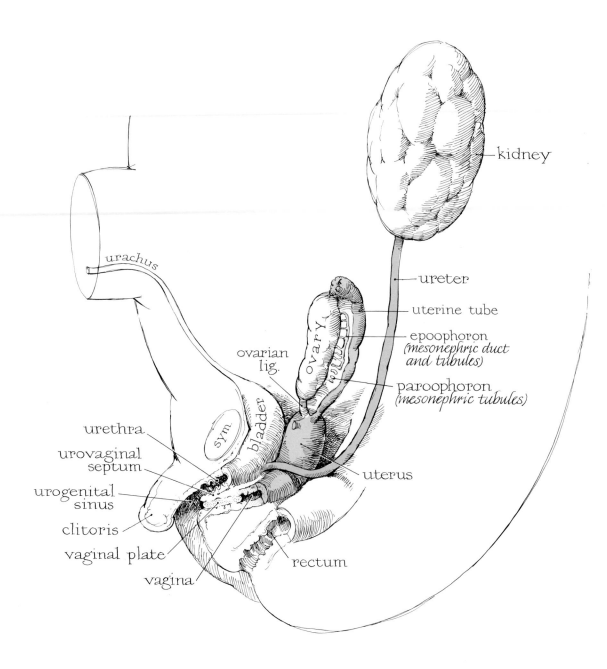

kidney

ureter

uterine tube

epoophoron
(mesonephric duct
and tubules)

paroophoron
(mesonephric tubules)

ovarian
lig.

ovary

urethra

urovaginal
septum

urogenital
sinus

clitoris

vaginal plate

vagina

bladder

sym.

urachus

uterus

rectum

Figure 24. Fetal period
78 mm   3 months
(108, 109, 110, 116)
The female urogenital system

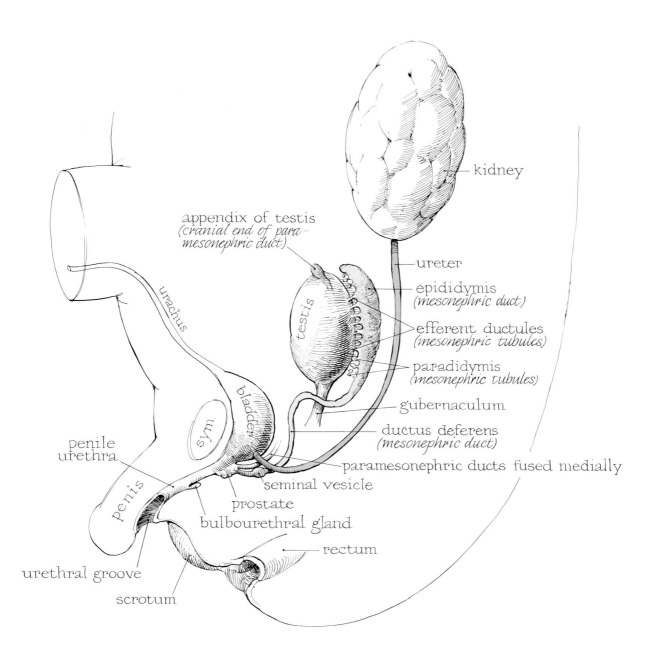

kidney

appendix of testis
(cranial end of para-
mesonephric duct)

ureter

epididymis
(mesonephric duct)

efferent ductules
(mesonephric tubules)

testis

paradidymis
(mesonephric tubules)

urachus

gubernaculum

ductus deferens
(mesonephric duct)

bladder

sym

paramesonephric ducts fused medially

penile
urethra

seminal vesicle

penis

prostate

bulbourethral gland

rectum

urethral groove

scrotum

Figure 25. Fetal period
78 mm   3 months
(106, 109, 111, 116)
The male urogenital system

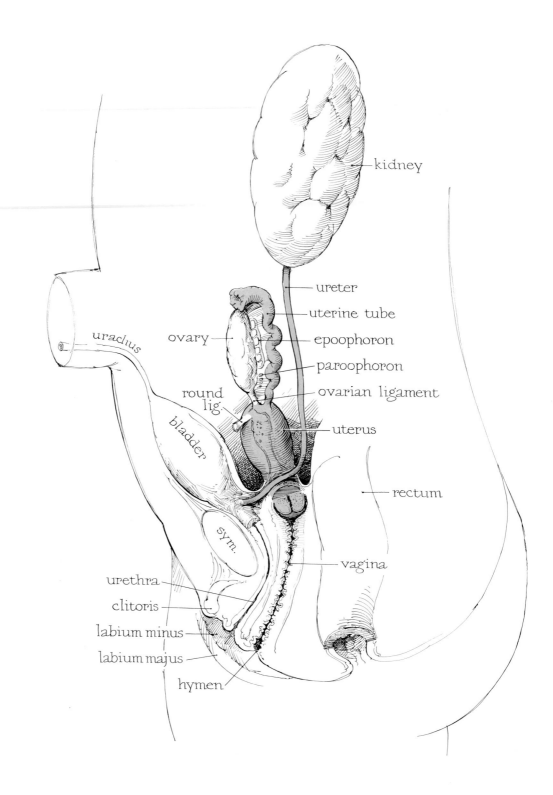

Figure 26. At term
(7, 9, 23, 108, 109, 110)
The female urogenital system

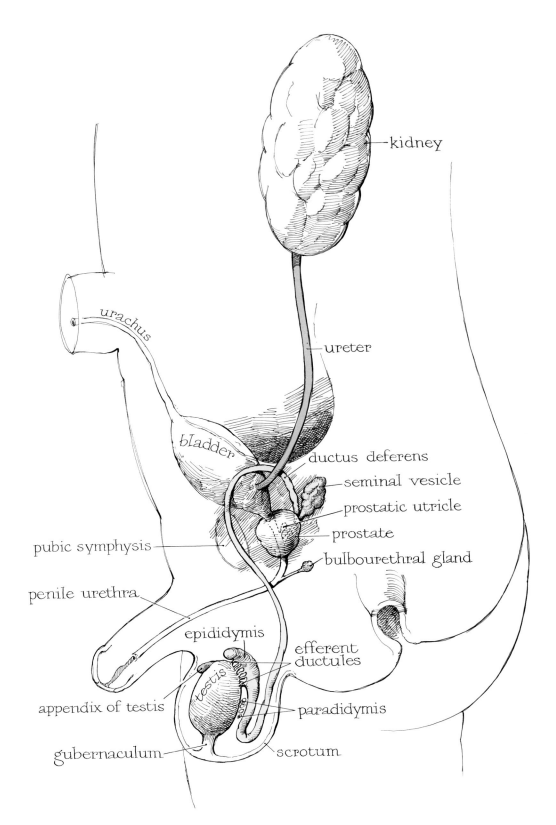

kidney

urachus

ureter

bladder

ductus deferens

seminal vesicle

prostatic utricle

prostate

bulbourethral gland

pubic symphysis

penile urethra

epididymis

efferent ductules

appendix of testis

testis

paradidymis

gubernaculum

scrotum

Figure 27. At term
(7, 9, 23)
The male urogenital system

The Heart

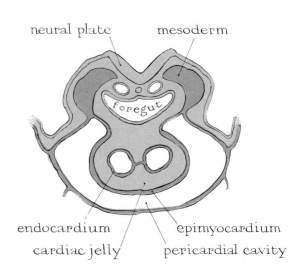

neural plate mesoderm

foregut

endocardial primordia
pericardial coelom

Development of the primitive heart tube

At the beginning of the fourth week paired *cardiac primordia* can be identified in the splanchnic mesoderm on either side of the foregut. As the embryo folds in the transverse plane, the primordia approach each other and fuse in the midline, forming a single *primitive heart tube* which consists of an inner layer termed the *endocardium* and an outer layer termed the *epimyocardium*.

The endocardium originates from mesenchyme. It is continuous with the endothelial lining of the blood vessels and will form the internal lining of the heart. The epimyocardium originates from splanchnic mesoderm. It will form the heart muscle and the epicardium (visceral pericardium). The parietal pericardium and the fibrous pericardium are derived from somatic mesoderm.

The primitive heart tube elongates rapidly and soon fills the pericardial cavity. As it does so it bends into an S shape. The primitive divisions of the heart can then be seen as a series of dilations separated by grooves. Named in order of blood flow, they are: the *sinus venosus* (paired), the *primitive atrium*, the *primitive ventricle*, the *bulbus cordis*, and the *truncus arteriosus*. About the middle of the fourth week the heart begins to beat and a primitive circulation is established to the central nervous system, the yolk sac, and the placenta.

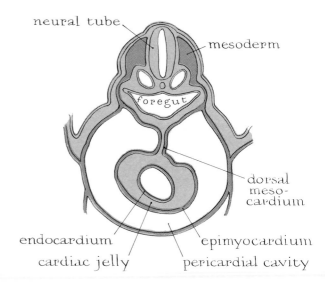

neural plate mesoderm

foregut

endocardium epimyocardium
cardiac jelly pericardial cavity

neural tube

mesoderm

foregut

dorsal meso-cardium

endocardium epimyocardium
cardiac jelly pericardial cavity

Late third and early fourth weeks
Top: *Stage 9*
Middle, bottom: *Stage 10*
(30, 49, 54, 58)
Fusion of the cardiac primordia as seen in transverse sections

60

The partition of the atrioventricular canal

The opening between the primitive atrium and the primitive ventricle is termed the *common atrioventricular canal*. Toward the end of the fourth week (stage 13) paired local thickenings of connective tissue termed the *dorsal* and *ventral endocardial cushions* develop in the walls of the common atrioventricular canal. They grow toward each other and about the beginning of the sixth week (stage 16) they meet and fuse, dividing the common atrioventricular canal into *right* and *left atrioventricular orifices*.

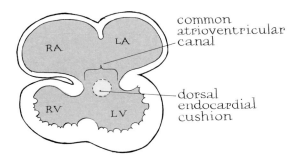

Stage 13   4 weeks (5)
Coronal section of the heart

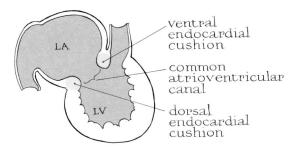

Stage 13   4 weeks (133)
Sagittal section of the heart

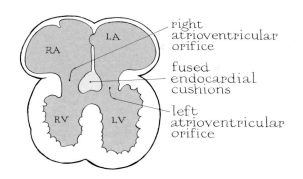

Stage 17   6th week (5)
Coronal section of the heart

The partition of the atrium

Two septa, termed the *septum primum* and the *septum secundum,* participate in dividing the primitive atrium into right and left chambers. The septum primum first appears during the fourth week (stage 12) as a crescent-shaped partition in the dorsocephalic wall of the primitive atrium. During the fifth and sixth weeks the septum primum grows toward the endocardial cushions. The opening between the caudal margin of the septum primum and the endocardial cushions is termed the *foramen primum.* It is a transient structure which is obliterated when the septum primum meets the fused endocardial cushions.

Just as the septum primum is about to contact the endocardial cushions a second opening termed the *foramen secundum* appears in the cranial part of the septum primum. It rapidly becomes larger and by the time the foramen primum closes during the sixth week (stage 17) the foramen secundum is large enough to allow most of the blood from the right atrium to pass directly into the left atrium.

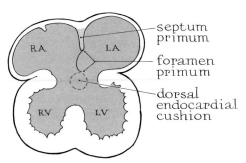
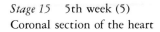

Stage 15 5th week (5)
Coronal section of the heart

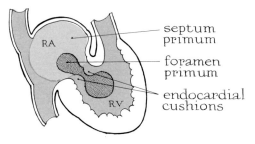

Stage 15 5th week (125)
Parasagittal section through the right atrium and ventricle

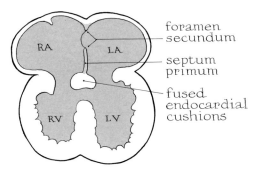

Stage 17 6th week (5)
Coronal section of the heart

62

During the seventh or eighth week a new interatrial partition termed the *septum secundum*
appears to the right of the septum primum.
The septum secundum grows toward the endocardial cushions in such a way that its crescent-
shaped free margin forms an oval opening
termed the *foramen ovale.* With continued
growth the foramen ovale becomes completely
covered by the septum primum, which acts as a
one-way valve allowing blood to flow from the
right atrium through the foramen ovale and the
foramen secundum into the left atrium. After
birth, the septum primum and the septum
secundum normally fuse to complete the
interatrial septum.

It should be noted that the septum secundum grows much more slowly than the septum
primum. The septum primum develops rapidly
between the fourth and sixth weeks (stages 12
to 17). In contrast, the septum secundum
makes its appearance sometime during the seventh or eighth week (stages 18 through 21) and
continues to develop until the latter part of the
fetal period.

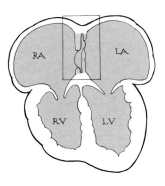

Fetal period (5)
Coronal section of the heart

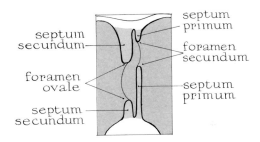

Fetal period
Coronal section of septum secundum and
septum primum

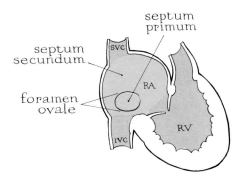

Fetal period (132)
Parasagittal section through the right
atrium and ventricle

The partition of the primitive ventricle

During the fourth week (stage 12) a partition termed the *muscular part of the interventricular septum* appears in the caudal part of the primitive ventricle. The opening which lies between this part of the septum and the endocardial cushions is termed the *interventricular foramen*.

During the fifth and sixth weeks the muscular part of the interventricular septum becomes larger, and in the seventh week (stage 18 or 19) the interventricular foramen is closed by connective tissue contributed by the interventricular septum, the right side of the fused endocardial cushions, and the bulbar ridges. This mass of connective tissue later becomes a fibrous sheet termed the *membranous part of the interventricular septum.* After the closure of the interventricular foramen, all the blood from the right ventricle passes into the pulmonary trunk and all the blood from the left ventricle passes into the aorta. Early in the fetal period the *right (tricuspid)* and *left (bicuspid) atrioventricular valves* arise from subendothelial tissue derived in part from the fused endocardial cushions and in part from adjacent connective tissue around the atrioventricular openings.

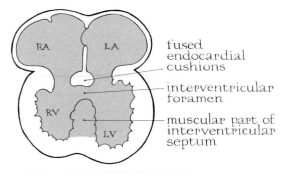

Stage 17   6th week (5)
Coronal section of the heart

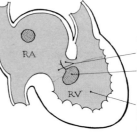

Stage 17   6th week (125)
Parasagittal section through the right atrium and ventricle

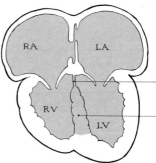

Fetal period (5)
Coronal section of the heart

The partition of the truncus arteriosus and the bulbus cordis

Early in the fifth week (stage 14) a pair of ridges forms in the truncus arteriosus between the roots of the fourth and sixth aortic arches. These ridges grow toward the right ventricle in a spiral pattern and extend into the bulbus cordis and the ventricle, where they are termed the *right* and *left bulbar ridges*. During the fifth and sixth weeks the ridges approach each other, and at stage 17 they fuse, forming a complete partition termed the *aorticopulmonary septum*. This divides the primitive lumen of the truncus arteriosus and the bulbus cordis into two channels: an *aortic channel*, which conveys blood from the left ventricle to the fourth aortic arches, and a *pulmonary channel*, which conveys blood from the right ventricle to the sixth aortic arches. After the formation of the aorticopulmonary septum, the aortic and pulmonary semilunar valves arise from proliferations of subendothelial tissue derived in part from the bulbar ridges and in part from interposed accessory ridges.

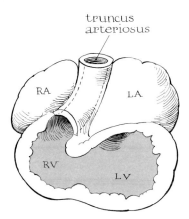

Stage 13 4 weeks (125)
Ventral view of the heart. The heart is dissected to expose the interior of the ventricular cavity.

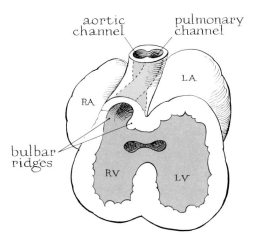

Stage 15 5th week (125)
Ventral view of the heart.

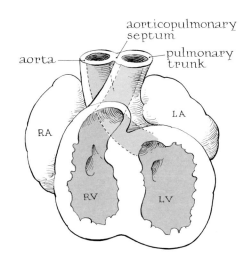

Stage 17 6th week (125)
Ventral view of the heart.

The fate of the sinus venosus

During the fourth week the sinus venosus receives blood from the common cardinal veins, the vitelline veins (via the hepatocardiac channels), and the umbilical veins. During the fifth week these veins undergo radical transformations and the sinus venosus is incorporated into the dorsal heart wall. The left horn of the sinus venosus and the proximal part of the left common cardinal vein form the coronary sinus. The right horn of the sinus venosus forms a portion of the dorsal wall of the right atrium. In the adult it can be seen as a smooth area, termed the *sinus venarum,* between the openings of the superior and inferior venae cavae.

The pulmonary veins

Toward the end of the fourth week (stage 13) angioblasts proliferate around the developing lung buds, and the primordium of the *common pulmonary vein* appears as a blind diverticulum in the dorsal wall of the left atrium. Within a day or two (stage 14) the common pulmonary vein forms anastomoses with a venous plexus around the lung buds, and by the end of the fifth week (stage 15) pulmonary circulation is well established. In subsequent development the common pulmonary vein and its branches are absorbed into the atrial wall with the result that there are at first two, and finally four separate openings of pulmonary veins into the left atrium.

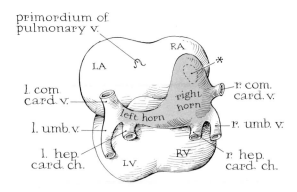

Stage 13   4 weeks (60)
Dorsal view of the heart.
The sinus venosus is shown in blue.
* Dotted lines indicate the opening
of the right horn of the sinus venosus
into the right atrium.

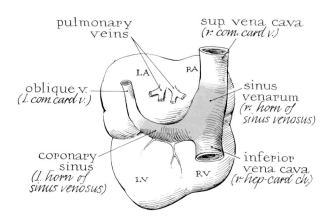

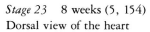

Stage 23   8 weeks (5, 154)
Dorsal view of the heart

66

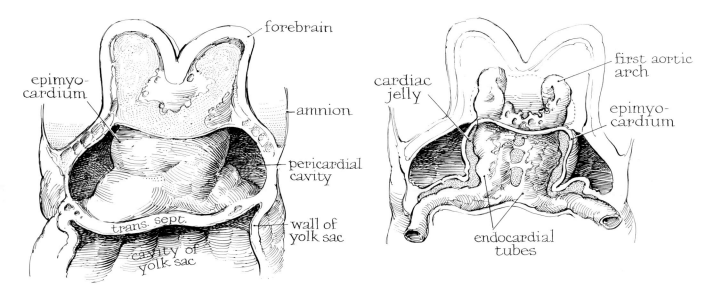

Figure 28. Stage 10
4 pairs of somites
(122)
Superficial dissection.
Ventral view.
The ventral body wall has been
removed to expose the pericardial
cavity and the epimyocardium.

Figure 29. Stage 10
4 pairs of somites
(122)
Deep dissection. Ventral view.
The ventral aspect of the
epimyocardium has been removed
to expose the right and left
endocardial tubes.

Figure 30. Stage 10
4 pairs of somites
(45, 58)
Transverse section

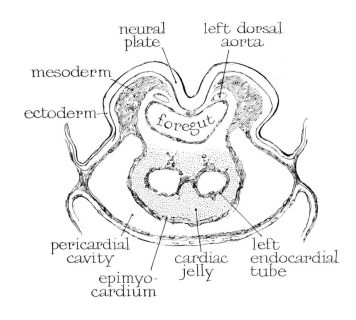

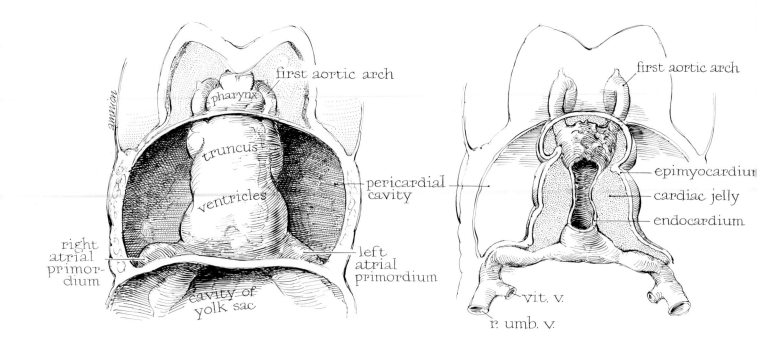

Figure 31. Stage 10
8 pairs of somites
(122)
Superficial dissection.
Ventral view.
The ventral body wall has been
removed to expose the pericardial
cavity and the epimyocardium.

Figure 32. Stage 10
8 pairs of somites
(122)
Deep dissection. Ventral view.
The epimyocardial layer has been
opened to reveal the endocardium.

Figure 33. Stage 10
8 pairs of somites
(54)
Transverse section

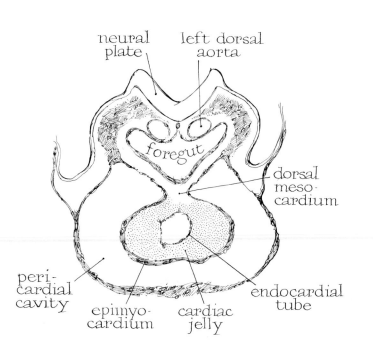

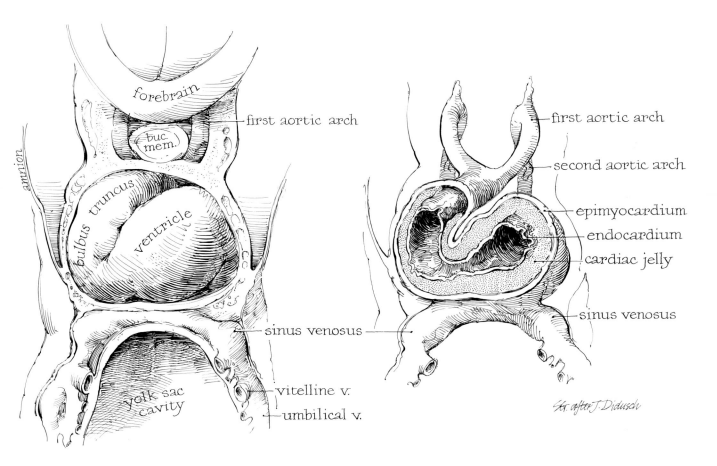

Figure 34. Stage 10
12 pairs of somites
(122)
Superficial dissection.
Ventral view.
The ventral body wall has been
removed to expose the pericardial
cavity and the epimyocardium.

Figure 35. Stage 10
12 pairs of somites
(122)
Deep dissection. Ventral view.
The epimyocardium has been cut
away to reveal the ventricular
part of the endocardial tube.

Figure 36. Stage 10
12 pairs of somites
(62)
Ventral view.
The endothelial portion of
the heart.

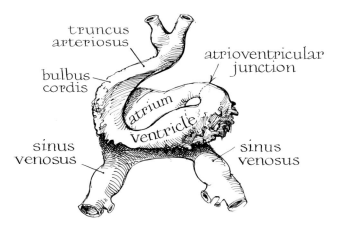

Figure 37. Stage 13
4–6 mm   28 days
30 or more pairs of somites
(62, 123, **125**, 134, 137)
Ventral view.
The heart is dissected to expose
the interior of the ventricular
cavity.

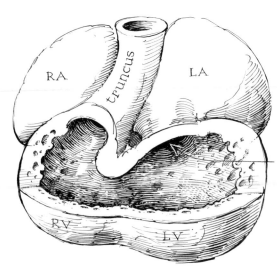

Figure 38. Stage 13
4–6 mm   28 days
30 or more pairs of somites
(**62**)
Ventral view.
The endothelial portion of
the heart.

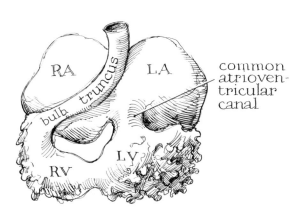

Figure 39. Stage 13
4–6 mm   28 days
30 or more pairs of somites
(4, 120, 123, 133, 134, 137)
Ventral view.
Further portions of the ventricle
are removed, as is the ventral
wall of the common atrial chamber.

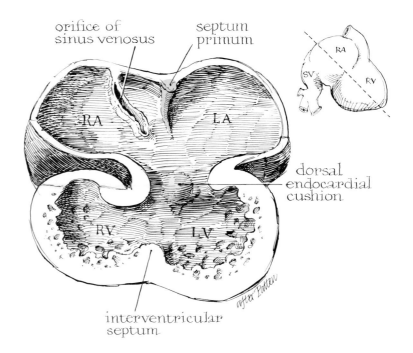

Figure 40. Stage 13
4–6 mm   28 days
30 or more pairs of somites
(61, 133, 134, 137)
Right lateral view.
Parasagittal section through the
right atrium and ventricle.

com. card.: right common cardinal vein
e: endocardial cushion
hep. card.: right hepato-
   cardiac channel
umb. v: right umbilical vein
s.v.: sinus venosus
2, 3, 4: aortic arches

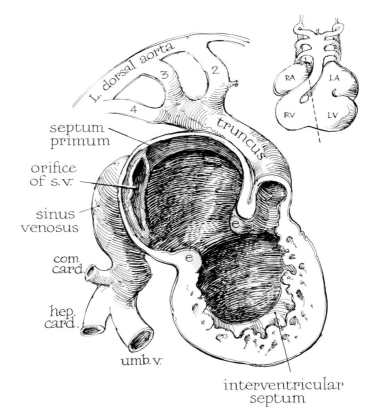

71

Figure 41. Stage 15
7–9 mm   33 days
(123, **125**, 134)
Ventral view.
The heart is dissected to expose
the interior of the ventricles.

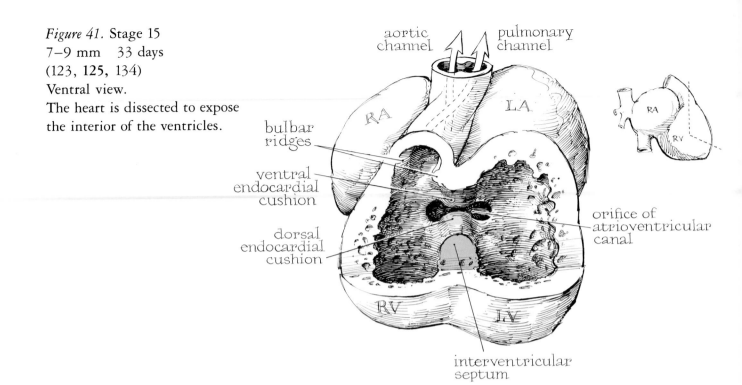

aortic
channel

pulmonary
channel

RA

L.A.

bulbar
ridges

ventral
endocardial
cushion

dorsal
endocardial
cushion

orifice of
atrioventicular
canal

RV

L.V.

interventricular
septum

RA

RV

Figure 42. Stage 15
(62)
Ventral view.
The endothelial portion of
the heart.

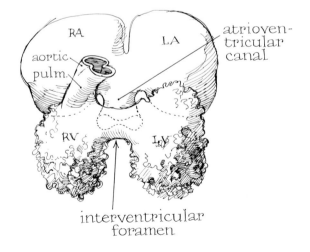

RA

LA

aortic
pulm.

atrioven-
tricular
canal

RV

L.V.

interventricular
foramen

Figure 43. Stage 15
7–9 mm   33 days
(**4**, 120, 133, 134)
Ventral view.
The ventral walls of both atria
and ventricles are removed.

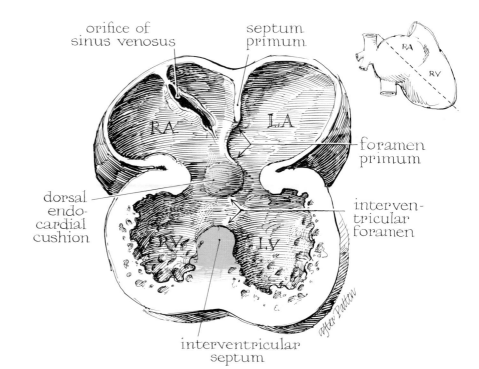

orifice of
sinus venosus

septum
primum

RA

LA

foramen
primum

dorsal
endo-
cardial
cushion

interven-
tricular
foramen

RV

LV

interventricular
septum

after Patten

Figure 44. Stage 15
7–9 mm   33 days
(**125**, 133, 134)
Right lateral view.
Parasagittal section through the
right atrium and ventricle.

com card: right common
    cardinal vein
dv: ductus venosus
e: endocardial cushion
F-1: foramen primum
hep card: right hepatocardiac
    channel
ic: internal carotid artery
postcard: postcardinal vein
precard: precardinal vein
s: opening of left horn
    of sinus venosus
Sept I: septum primum
sub: subclavian vein
3, 4, 6: aortic arches

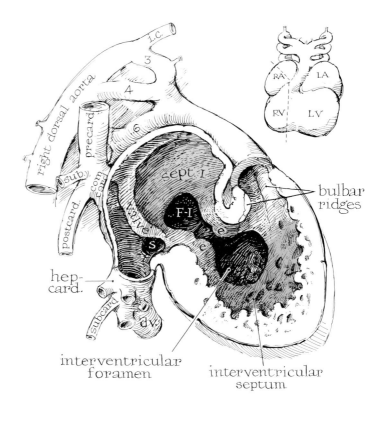

i.c.

3

right dorsal aorta

4

precard.

6

RA

LA

RV

LV

sub.

com card.

postcard.

sept. I

F-1

valve

e

bulbar
ridges

s

hep-
card.

subcard.

dv.

interventricular
foramen

interventricular
septum

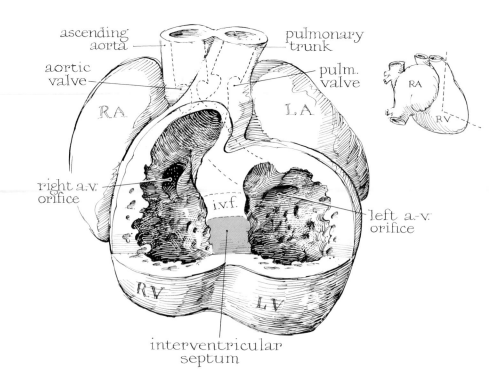

Figure 45. Stage 17
11–14 mm   41 days
(120, **125,** 133, 134, 135, 137)
Ventral view.
The heart is dissected to expose
the interior of the ventricles.

av: atrioventricular
ivf: interventricular foramen

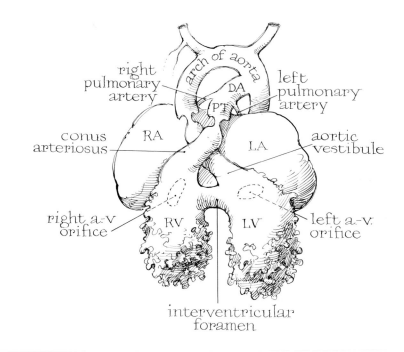

Figure 46. Stage 17
11–14 mm   41 days
(62)
Ventral view.
The endothelial portion
of the heart.

av: atrioventricular
DA: ductus arteriosus
PT: pulmonary trunk

Figure 47. Stage 17
11–14 mm   41 days
(120, **131**, 133, 135, 137)
Ventral view.
The ventral walls of both atria
and ventricles are removed.

endo cush: fused endocardial cushions
s: opening of left horn of
   sinus venosus
IVF: interventricular foramen

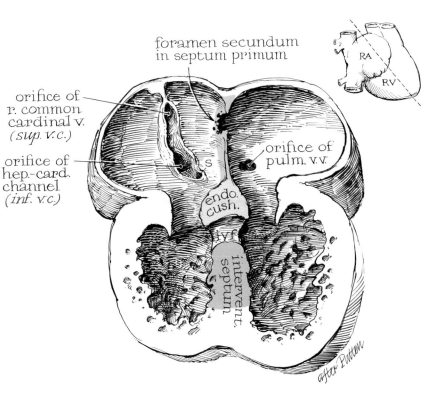

Figure 48. Stage 17
11–14 mm   41 days
(**125**, 131, 133, 135, 137)
Right lateral view.
Parasagittal section through the
right atrium and ventricle.

DA: ductus arteriosus
dv: ductus venosus
e: endocardial cushion
F-2: foramen secundum
pa: pulmonary artery
postcard: postcardinal vein
PT: pulmonary trunk
s: opening of left horn of
   sinus venosus
subcl: subclavian vein
supra: supracardinal vein
valve: left venous valve

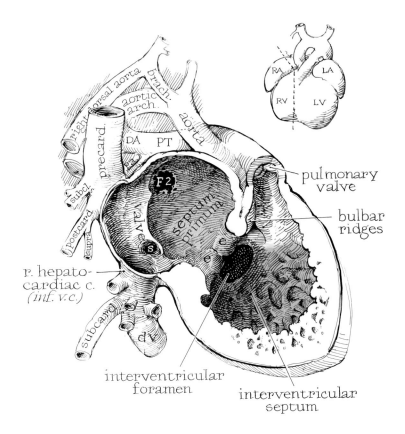

Figure 49. Stage 23
27–31 mm   56 days
(9, 24, 126)
Ventral view.
The heart is dissected to expose
the interior of the ventricles.

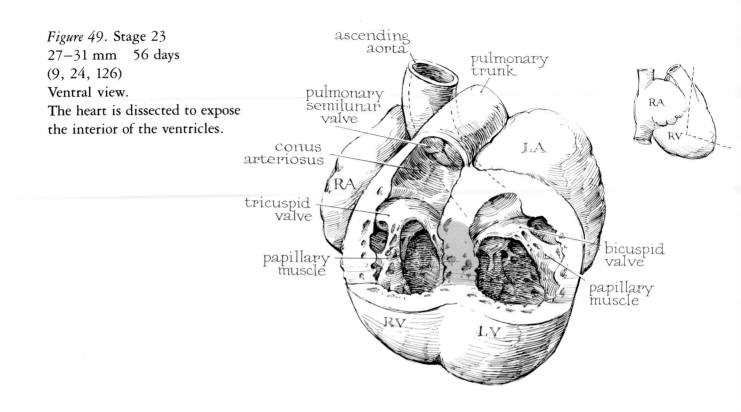

Figure 50. Stage 23
27–31 mm   56 days
(9, 24, 126)
The endothelial portion of
the heart

av: atrioventricular
DA: ductus arteriosus
PT: pulmonary trunk

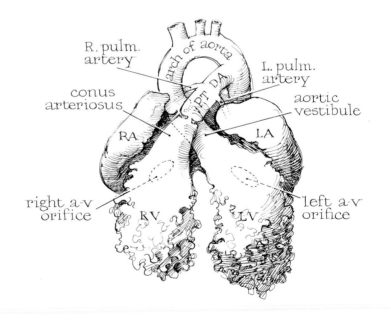

Figure 51. Stage 23
27–31 mm   56 days
(**4**, 26, 121, 126)
Ventral view.
The ventral walls of both atria
and ventricles are removed.

b: dorsal cusp of bicuspid
   valve
L: left venous valve
S: orifice of coronary sinus
SV: sinus venarum

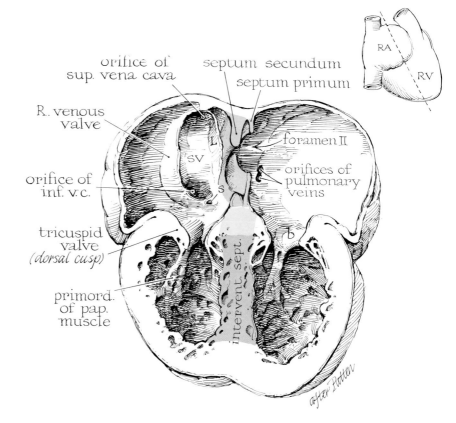

orifice of
sup. vena cava

septum secundum
septum primum

R. venous
valve

foramen II

orifices of
pulmonary
veins

orifice of
inf. v.c.

tricuspid
valve
(*dorsal cusp*)

primord.
of pap.
muscle

intervent. sept.

b

after Patten

Figure 52. Stage 23
27–31 mm   56 days
(11, 24, **126**)
Right lateral view.
Parasagittal section through the
right atrium and ventricle.

IVC: inferior vena cava
Sept. II: septum secundum
SVC: superior vena cava
v: valve of coronary sinus

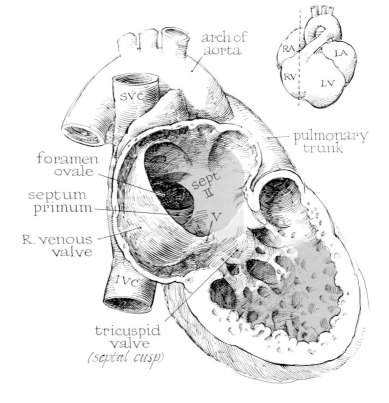

arch of
aorta

SVC

pulmonary
trunk

foramen
ovale

sept.
II

V

septum
primum

R. venous
valve

IVC

tricuspid
valve
(*septal cusp*)

Figure 53. Fetal period
(4, 7, 11, 23)
Ventral view.
The ventral walls of the atria
and the ventricles are removed.

b: dorsal cusp of bicuspid
   valve
m: membranous portion of
   interventricular septum
v: valve of coronary sinus

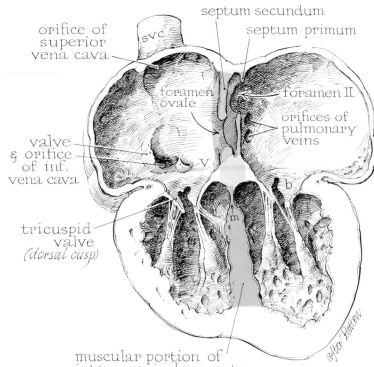

Figure 54. Fetal period
(7, 11, 23, 132)
Right lateral view.
Parasagittal section through the
right atrium and ventricle.

b: brachiocephalic trunk
c: left common carotid artery
ivc: inferior vena cava
s: left subclavian artery
svc: superior vena cava

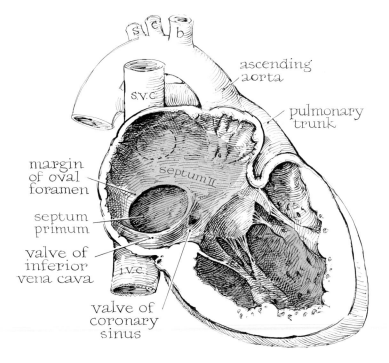

The Arteries

The early development of blood vessels

Blood vessels and blood cells develop from mesoderm. Late in the third week isolated areas of endothelial tissue appear and unite to form plexuses within which channels develop and enlarge to form primitive arteries and veins. Subsequently connective tissue and smooth muscle components of the blood vessels develop from adjacent mesenchyme.

The arteries in the fourth week

The primitive arterial pattern is established early in the fourth week. Ventral to the foregut the truncus arteriosus expands to form the *aortic sac,* from which paired right and left *first aortic arches* pass dorsally and then turn caudally as the *right* and *left dorsal aortae.* Each dorsal aorta gives off numerous *ventral segmental arteries* to the yolk sac, and *dorsal intersegmental arteries* to the neural tube and body wall. Near the connecting stalk each dorsal aorta breaks up into a plexus which communicates with the umbilical artery.

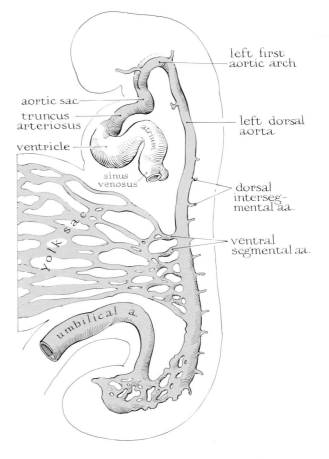

Stage 11 4th week (60, 141)
Lateral view of the primitive arterial pattern. For the sake of simplicity paired arteries are shown on the left side only.

The aortic sac: The aortic sac is a broad arterial channel distal to the truncus arteriosus. All of the aortic arches take origin from the aortic sac, and the sac itself makes a substantial contribution to the pulmonary trunk, the definitive arch of the aorta, the brachiocephalic artery, and the common carotid arteries.* It should be stressed, however, that the boundaries of the aortic sac and the individual aortic arches are lost during embryonic development and that there are no exact landmarks to define the limits of the embryonic components in the adult arterial pattern.

The aortic arches

The significance of the aortic arches in the human embryo can best be understood by comparing them to homologous structures in lower vertebrates. In most embryonic fishes six pairs of aortic arches convey blood from the ventral aorta to the dorsal aortae. In most adult fishes derivatives of the first and second aortic arches supply structures in the head, while arches 3, 4, 5, and 6 supply the gills. In human embryos, however, the fifth pair of arches is vestigial or absent, and the remaining five pairs are never all clearly defined at one time because the first two pairs begin to degenerate as the others develop.

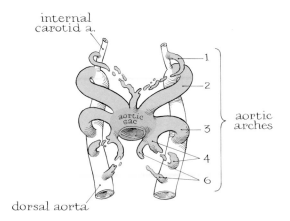

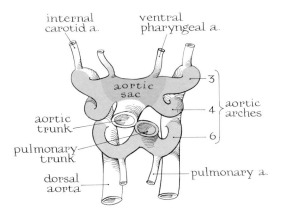

Stage 16   6th week   (141)
Ventral view of the third, fourth, and sixth aortic arches. The first and second arches have degenerated. Their remnants are seen here as the right and left ventral pharyngeal arteries, which will form the proximal parts of the external carotid arteries.

*Phylogenetically, the common carotid arteries have evolved from the ventral stems of the third aortic arches. In human embryos, however, the ventral aortic stems are represented by the aortic sac and there is "no justification for the use of the term *ventral aortae* in man, since such vessels are not to be found at any stage of his development" (Congdon 1922 [141]).

The fate of the aortic arches may be summarized as follows:

1 and 2. The first and second pairs of arches contribute to the formation of a plexus which subsequently gives rise to the external carotid artery and its branches.

3. The third pair of arches contributes to the formation of the proximal part of the internal carotid arteries.

4. The left fourth aortic arch contributes to a small part of the definitive arch of the aorta. The right fourth aortic arch contributes to the proximal part of the right subclavian artery.

5. Anomalous vessels, thought to be vestiges of the fifth pair of arches, are sometimes found in human embryos.

6. The pulmonary arteries arise as outgrowths of the sixth aortic arches. The right sixth aortic arch distal to the origin of the pulmonary artery degenerates. The left sixth aortic arch distal to the origin of the pulmonary artery persists throughout fetal life as the *ductus arteriosus,* and can be identified in the adult as the *ligamentum arteriosum.*

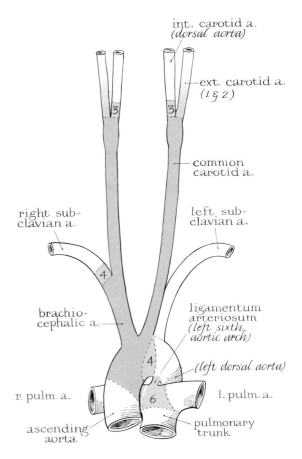

Adult (138)
The definitive arch of the aorta and the pulmonary arteries in the adult. The contributions of the aortic arches are indicated by numbers. The names of other embryonic components are in italics. The orange area indicates the contribution of the aortic sac.

The aorta

During the fourth week the paired dorsal aortae caudal to the tenth dorsal intersegmental artery fuse to form the *descending aorta*. Cranial to the tenth intersegmental artery the right and left dorsal aortae persist until the seventh week, when the definitive arterial pattern is established. At this time the part of the right dorsal aorta caudal to the origin of the primitive subclavian artery degenerates and the remaining part of the right dorsal aorta, together with a remnant of the right fourth aortic arch, takes part in the formation of the right subclavian artery. The cranial portion of the left dorsal aorta persists and forms part of the definitive arch of the aorta, which also includes contributions from the truncus arteriosus, the aortic sac, the left fourth aortic arch, and a short portion of the fused dorsal aortae.

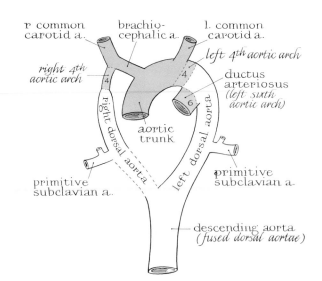

Stage 18 7th week (138, 141)
The right and left dorsal aortae early in the seventh week. Dotted lines indicate the portion of the right dorsal aorta, which degenerates about the middle of the seventh week.

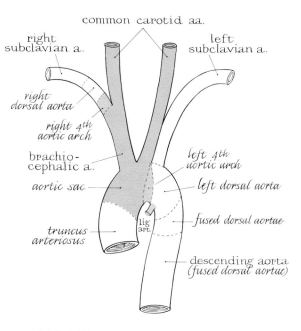

Adult (138)
The definitive arch of the aorta in the adult. The names of embryonic components are indicated in italics.

Branches of the descending aorta

The descending aorta gives off three series of branches: (1) *ventral segmental arteries,* which supply the yolk sac, the gut, and the fetal part of the placenta, (2) *lateral segmental arteries,* which principally supply the urogenital system, and (3) *dorsal intersegmental arteries,* which supply the body wall and the spinal cord.

Ventral segmental arteries

During the fourth week the original number of ventral segmental arteries to the yolk sac and the gut becomes greatly reduced through fusion and degeneration, with the result that only three major arteries remain. They are: (1) the *celiac artery,* which supplies the foregut, (2) the *superior mesenteric artery,* which supplies the midgut and continues distally as the *vitelline artery,* to the yolk sac, and (3) the *inferior mesenteric artery,* which supplies the hindgut. In the thoracic region the esophageal and bronchial arteries are also derived from ventral segmental arteries.

The *umbilical arteries,* which convey blood from the dorsal aortae to the placenta, are specialized members of the ventral segmental series. Shortly after the paired dorsal aortae fuse, the stem of the umbilical artery on each side degenerates and a new stem forms via an anastomosis with the fifth lumbar dorsal intersegmental artery. This new stem persists as the common iliac artery and gives off branches which become the external and internal iliac arteries. In the adult, the derivative of the umbilical artery is seen as a branch of the internal iliac. It gives off one or more superior vesical arteries to the bladder and then continues as a fibrous cord termed the *lateral umbilical ligament,* which lies on the inner surface of the ventral abdominal wall and extends to the umbilicus.

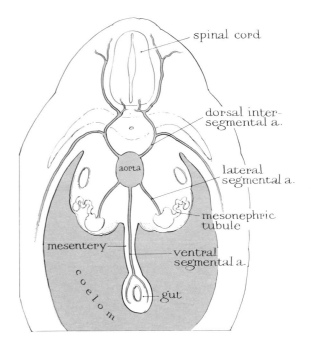

Stage 16   6th week (5, 8)
Schematic transverse section through the mid-thoracic region

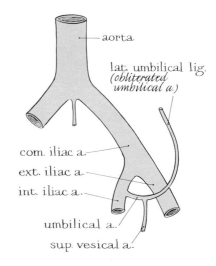

Adult (144)
Derivatives of the fifth lumbar dorsal intersegmental artery and the umbilical artery as seen in the adult

Lateral segmental arteries

The *lateral segmental* branches of the aorta are paired vessels which supply the mesonephroi, the metanephroi, the suprarenal glands, the gonads, and the diaphragm. They give rise to the renal, testicular or ovarian, middle suprarenal, and phrenic arteries of the adult.

Dorsal intersegmental arteries

The aorta gives off thirty or more pairs of *dorsal intersegmental arteries* between somites. In the cervical region the vertebral artery originates from anastomoses between the first six dorsal intersegmental arteries. The seventh pair of dorsal intersegmental arteries contributes to the formation of the subclavian arteries. In the thoracic and abdominal regions, dorsal intersegmental arteries give rise to the posterior intercostal arteries and the lumbar arteries, respectively. As noted previously, the fifth lumbar dorsal intersegmental artery takes part in the formation of the arteries of the pelvis and the lower limbs.

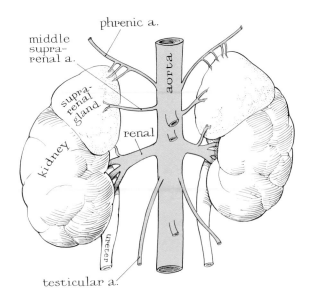

Infant (1, 7, 23)
Derivatives of the lateral segmental arteries as seen at birth

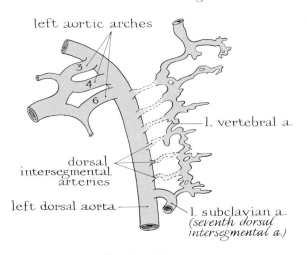

Stage 16 6th week (141, 143)
The vertebral artery early in the sixth week. Degenerating portions of dorsal intersegmental arteries are indicated by dotted lines.

Table 5. The Arteries (11, 138)

Embryonic structure	Adult structure
Aortic sac	Contributes to pulmonary trunk; definitive arch of aorta, brachio-cephalic a., common carotid aa.
Aortic arches:	
1, 2	Contribute to external carotid a.
3	Proximal part of internal carotid a.
4	*Left:* contributes to definitive arch of aorta. *Right:* proximal part of right subclavian a.
5	Vestigial or absent
6	Contribute to pulmonary trunk and pulmonary aa.
Left 6th arch: ductus arteriosus	Ligamentum arteriosum
Dorsal aortae	Fuse to form descending aorta. Right dorsal aorta contributes to right subclavian a.; left dorsal aorta contributes to arch of aorta.
Branches of descending aorta:	
Ventral segmental aa.	Celiac a.; superior mesenteric a.; inferior mesenteric a.
Umbilical aa.	Lateral umbilical ligaments
Lateral segmental aa.	Renal aa.; testicular or ovarian aa.; middle suprarenal aa.; phrenic aa.
Dorsal intersegmental aa.	Vertebral aa.; contribute to subclavian aa.; posterior intercostal aa.; lumbar aa.; contribute to aa. of pelvis and leg

Figure 55. Stage 12
3–5 mm   26 days
21–29 pairs of somites
(32, 60, 141)
Left lateral view of the arteries.
Paired vessels are shown only on
the left.

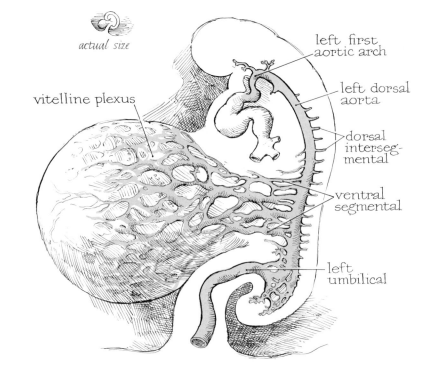

actual size

left first
aortic arch

left dorsal
aorta

dorsal
interseg-
mental

vitelline plexus

ventral
segmental

left
umbilical

Figure 56. Stage 12
3–5 mm   26 days
21–29 pairs of somites
(32, 60, 141)
Ventral view of the aortic arches

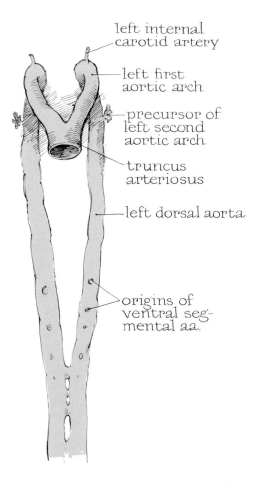

left internal
carotid artery

left first
aortic arch

precursor of
left second
aortic arch

truncus
arteriosus

left dorsal aorta

origins of
ventral seg-
mental aa.

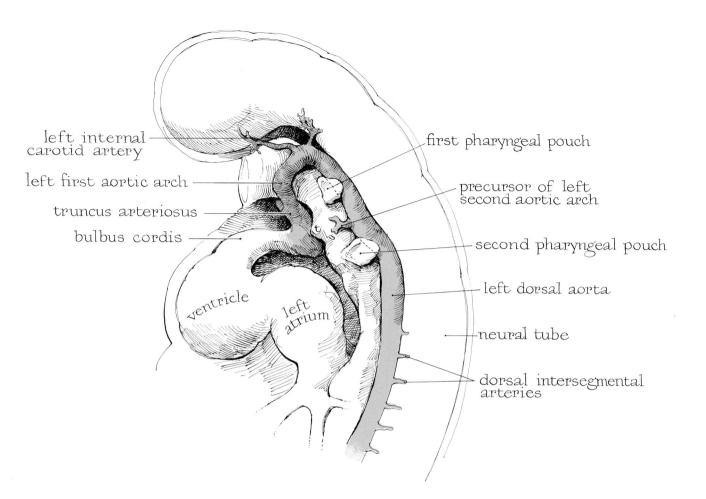

left internal carotid artery

left first aortic arch

truncus arteriosus

bulbus cordis

ventricle

left atrium

first pharyngeal pouch

precursor of left second aortic arch

second pharyngeal pouch

left dorsal aorta

neural tube

dorsal intersegmental arteries

Figure 57. Stage 12
3–5 mm   26 days
21–29 pairs of somites
(32, 100, 104, 141, 142, 143)
Left lateral view of the aortic arches

t: thyroid diverticulum

Figure 58. Stage 13
4–6 mm   28 days
30 or more pairs of somites
(61)
Left lateral view of the arteries

* unpaired midline artery

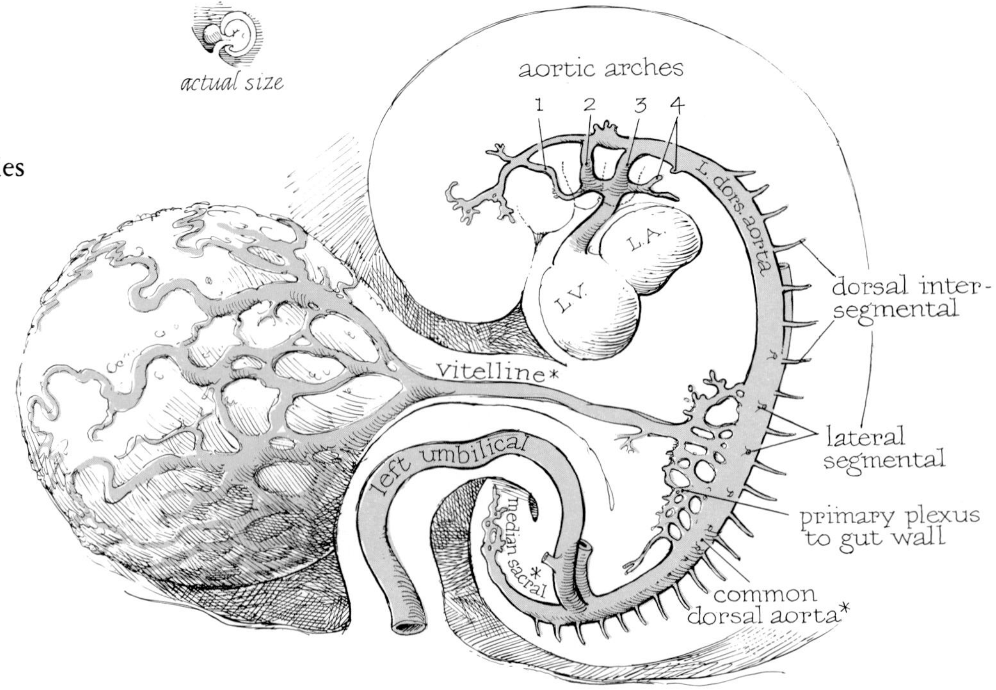

actual size

aortic arches
1 2 3 4

L. dors. aorta

L.V.   L.A.

vitelline*

dorsal inter-
segmental

lateral
segmental

primary plexus
to gut wall

left umbilical

median sacral*

common
dorsal aorta*

Figure 59. Stage 13
4–6 mm   28 days
30 or more pairs of somites
(141)
Ventral view of the aortic arches

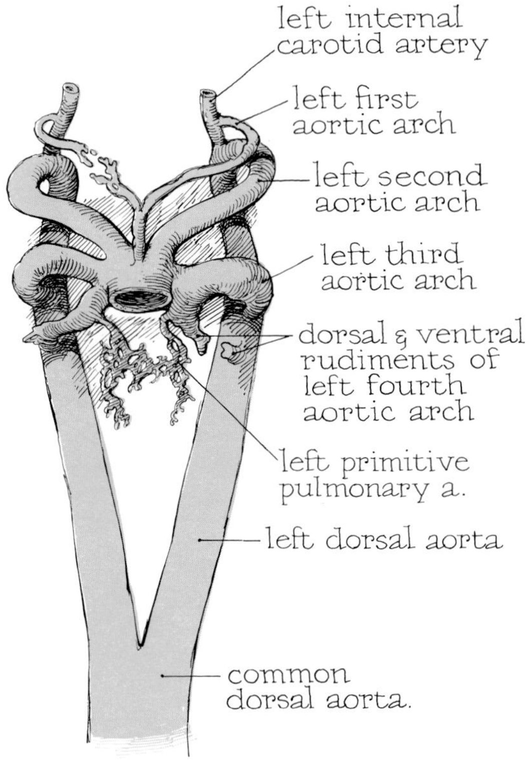

left internal
carotid artery

left first
aortic arch

left second
aortic arch

left third
aortic arch

dorsal & ventral
rudiments of
left fourth
aortic arch

left primitive
pulmonary a.

left dorsal aorta

common
dorsal aorta.

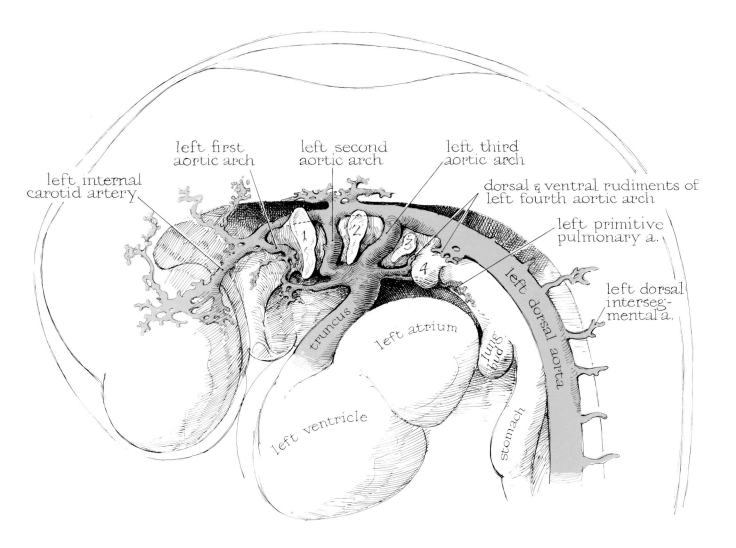

Figure 60. Stage 13
4–6 mm   28 days
30 or more pairs of somites
(61, 100, 103, 123, 141, 142, 143)
Lateral view of the aortic arches

1, 2, 3, 4: pharyngeal pouches

Figure 61. Stage 14
5–7 mm   32 days
(61)
Left lateral view of the arteries

* unpaired midline artery

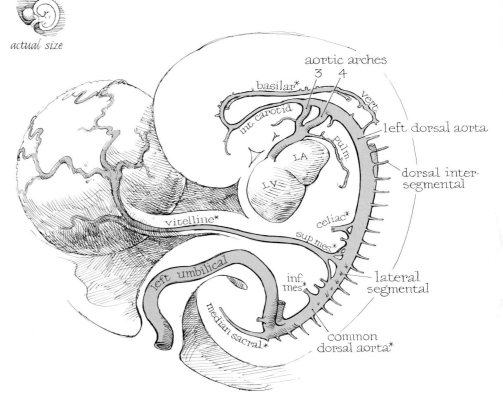

Figure 62. Stage 14
5–7 mm   32 days
(141)
Ventral view of the aortic arches

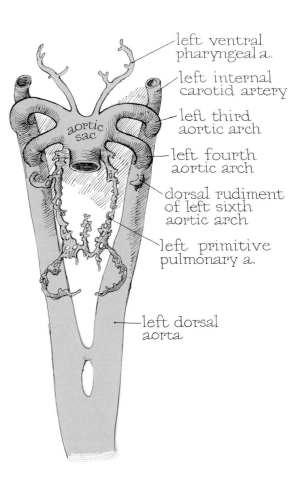

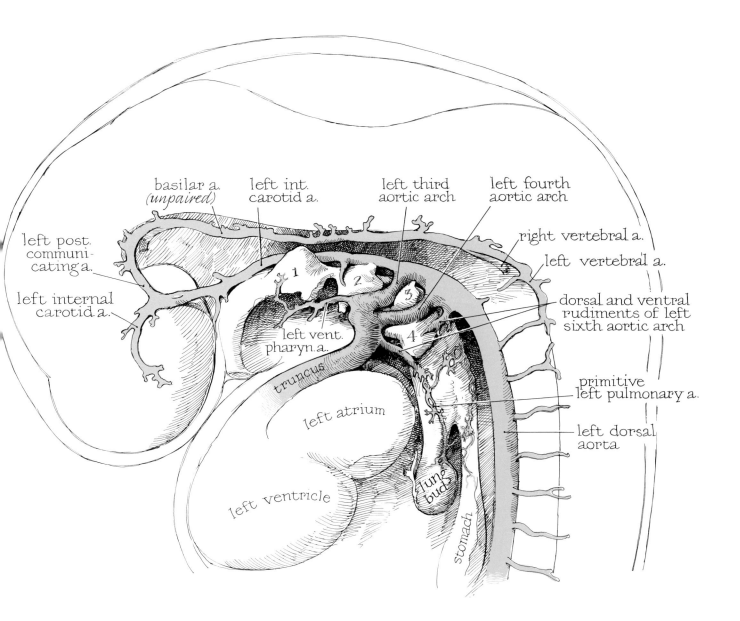

Figure 63. Stage 14
5–7 mm   32 days
(61, 100, 103, 123, 141, 142, 143)
Left lateral view of the aortic arches

1, 2, 3, 4: pharyngeal pouches

Figure 64. Stage 16
8–11 mm   37 days
(62)
Left lateral view of the arteries

* unpaired midline artery

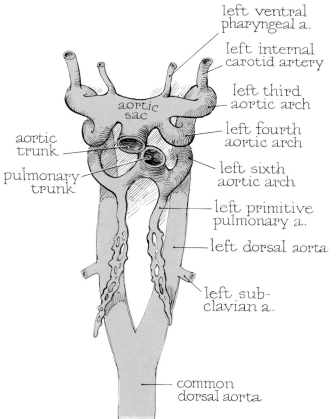

actual size

aortic arches

basilar*

int. carotid

vertebral

3 4 6

left dorsal aorta

LA

pulm.

LV

subclavian

common dorsal aorta*

vitelline*

celiac*

left umbilical

sup. mes.*

dorsal inter-segmental

inf. mes.*

lateral segmental

median sacral*

Figure 65. Stage 16
8–11 mm   37 days
(141)
Ventral view of the aortic arches

left ventral pharyngeal a.

left internal carotid artery

aortic sac

left third aortic arch

left fourth aortic arch

aortic trunk

left sixth aortic arch

pulmonary trunk

left primitive pulmonary a.

left dorsal aorta

left sub-clavian a.

common dorsal aorta

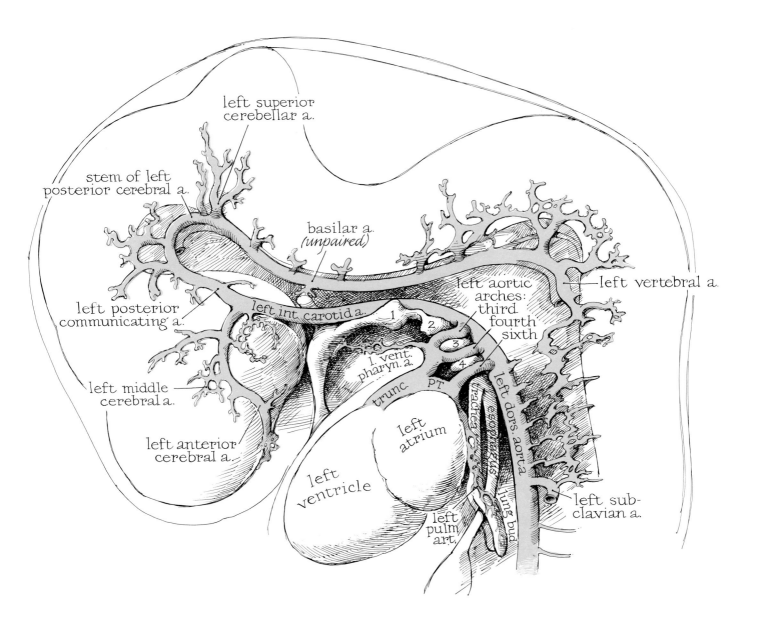

Figure 66. Stage 16
8–11 mm   37 days
(62, 100, 103, 141, 142, 143)
Left lateral view of the aortic arches

1, 2, 3, 4: pharyngeal pouches

Figure 67. Stage 18
13–17 mm   44 days
(62)
Left lateral view of the arteries

* unpaired midline artery

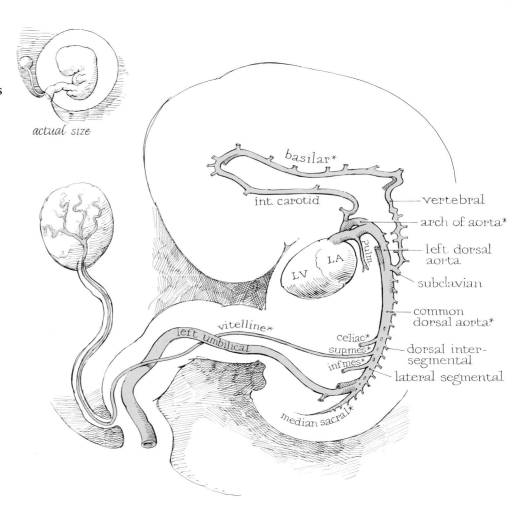

actual size

Figure 68. Stage 18
13–17 mm   44 days
(138, 141)
Ventral view of the aortic arches

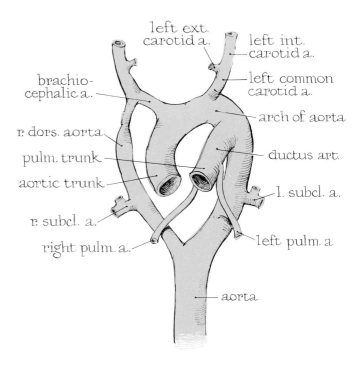

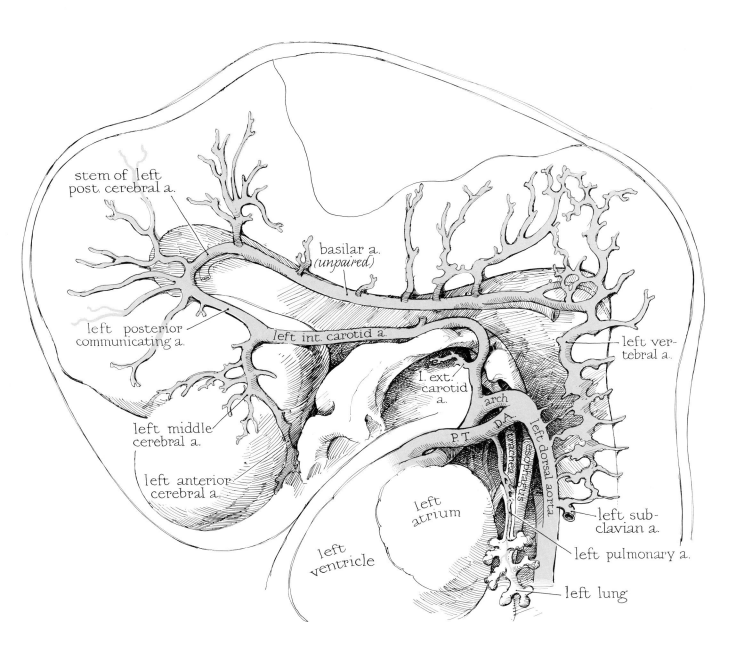

Figure 69. Stage 18
13–17 mm   44 days
(100, 103, 138, 141, 142, 143)
Left lateral view of the aortic arches

DA: ductus arteriosus
PT: pulmonary trunk

Figure 70. Stage 19
16–18 mm   48 days
(63, 66)
Left lateral view of the arteries

* unpaired midline artery

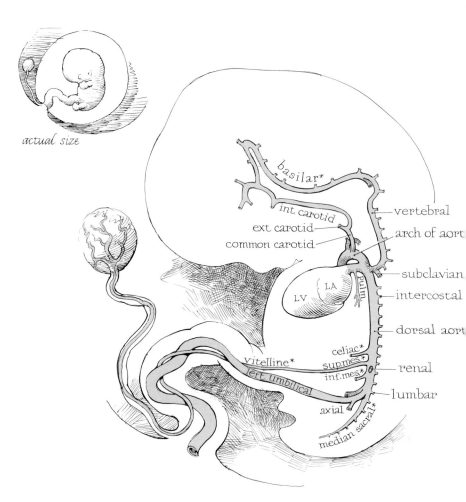

actual size

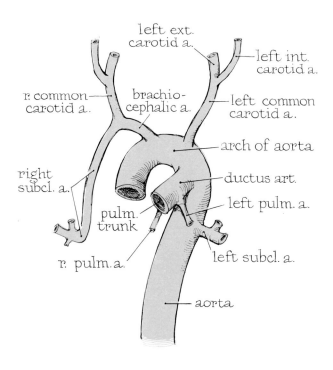

Figure 71. Stage 19
16–18 mm   48 days
(138, 141)
The aortic arches, ventral view

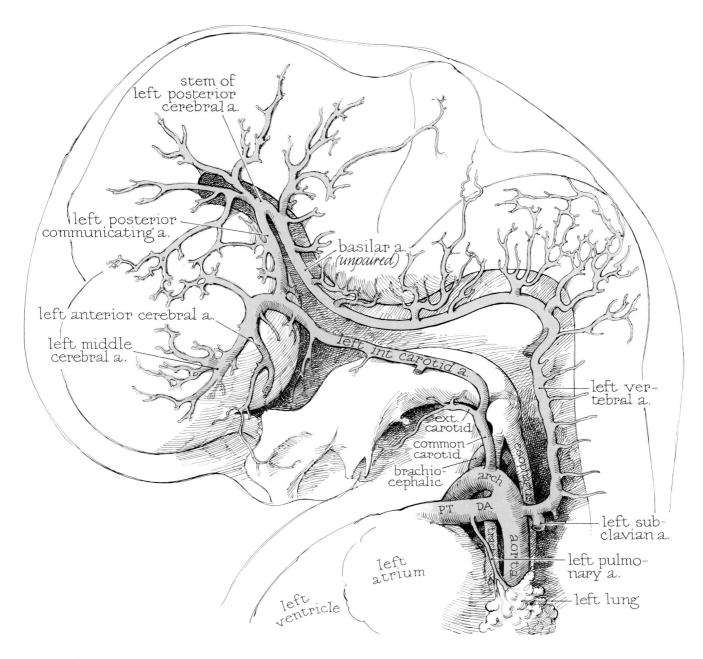

Figure 72. Stage 19
16–18 mm   48 days
(66, 138, 141, 142, 143)
Left lateral view of the aortic arches

DA: ductus arteriosus
PT: pulmonary trunk

The Veins

The veins in the fourth week

The primitive venous system consists of three sets of symmetrical paired veins: the *vitelline veins,* which return blood from the yolk sac and the gut; the *umbilical veins,* which return blood from the placenta; and the *precardinal* and *postcardinal veins,* which return blood from the head and the trunk. Near the heart the precardinal and postcardinal veins unite to form the *common cardinal veins,* which join the sinus venosus together with the vitelline and umbilical veins.

The vitelline veins

By the anastomosis of some parts and the atrophy of others, the right and left vitelline veins form the *portal vein* and its tributaries. The proximal portion of the right vitelline vein persists as the part of the *vena cava* which extends from the liver to the heart.

The umbilical veins

During the fifth week the right umbilical vein and the proximal portion of the left umbilical vein degenerate. At the same time, the left umbilical vein forms anastomoses with the hepatic sinusoids and a newly formed channel, termed the *ductus venosus,* conveys blood from the umbilical vein and the portal vein to the inferior vena cava and the sinus venosus. In the adult a remnant of the left umbilical vein persists as the *round ligament of the liver,* and a remnant of the ductus venosus persists as the *ligamentum venosum.*

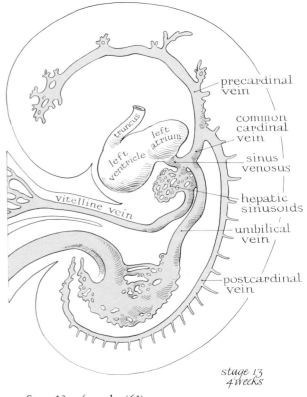

Stage 13 4 weeks (61)
Lateral view of the primitive venous system. For the sake of simplicity paired veins are shown on the left side only.

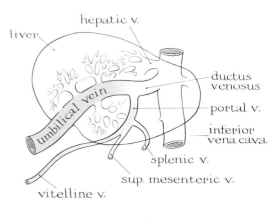

Stage 19 7th week (149)
Lateral view of the liver and associated veins late in the seventh week

The precardinal veins

The precardinal veins become the internal jugular veins and early in the eighth week the left brachiocephalic vein forms a connection between them. The left common cardinal vein then atrophies, and blood from the left internal jugular vein passes via the left brachiocephalic vein to the superior vena cava, which is formed by the right common cardinal vein and the proximal part of the right precardinal vein.

The postcardinal veins

During the seventh week the postcardinal veins begin to atrophy and soon disappear almost completely. The venous drainage of the trunk and legs is then taken over by a complex secondary system of veins consisting of the *subcardinals,* the *sacrocardinals,* and the *supracardinals* (see figs. 81–84).

The abdominal portion of the inferior vena cava is derived from the right sacrocardinal vein and the right subcardinal vein. The part of the inferior vena cava which lies dorsal to the liver is derived from an anastomosis between the right subcardinal vein and the right vitelline vein, and the portion of the inferior vena cava which conveys blood from the liver to the heart is derived from the persisting proximal portion of the right vitelline vein.

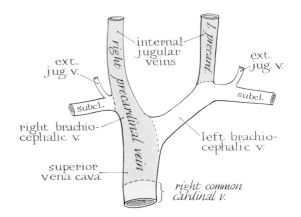

Adult (154)
The superior vena cava and its tributaries in the adult. A number of smaller veins are omitted for the sake of simplicity. Embryonic components are indicated in italics.

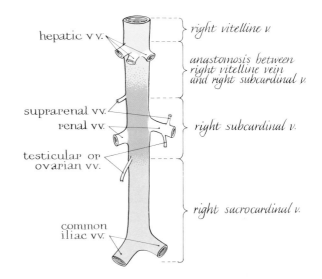

Adult (148)
The inferior vena cava in the adult. Embryonic components are indicated in italics.

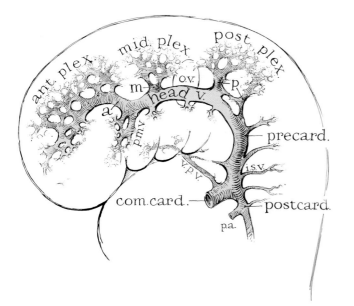

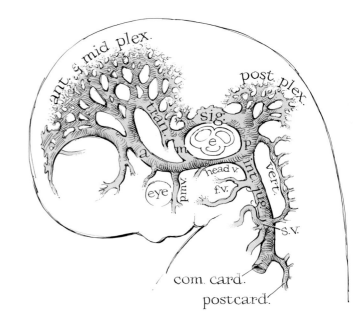

Figure 73. Stage 13
4–6 mm   28 days
30 or more pairs of somites
(61, 145, 153, 154, 155)
The precardinal vein and its
tributaries

a: stem of anterior cerebral
  plexus
isv: intersegmental vein
m: stem of middle cerebral
  plexus
ov: otic vesicle
p: stem of posterior cerebral
  plexus
pa: primitive vein of arm bud
pmv: primitive maxillary vein
vpv: ventral pharyngeal vein

Figure 74. Stage 19
16–18 mm   48 days
(145, 153, 154, 155)
The internal jugular vein and its
tributaries

a: stem of anterior cerebral
  plexus
e: internal ear
fv: facial vein
m: stem of middle cerebral
  plexus
p: stem of posterior cerebral
  plexus
pmv: primitive maxillary vein
sig: sigmoid sinus
sv: primitive subclavian vein
tran: primitive transverse sinus

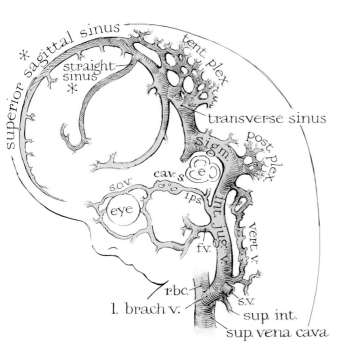

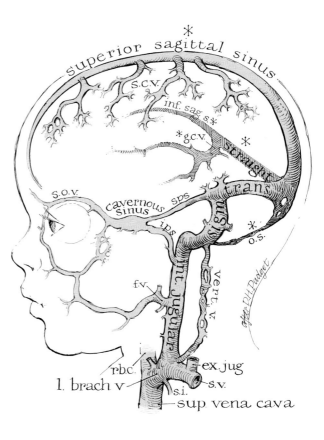

Figure 75. Early fetal period
40 mm   9 weeks
(153, 154, 155)
The internal jugular vein and its
tributaries

cav s: cavernous sinus
e: internal ear
fv: facial vein
ips: inferior petrosal sinus
1 brach v: left brachiocephalic
   vein
rbc: right brachicephalic vein
sigm: sigmoid sinus
sov: superior ophthalmic vein
sup int: left superior intercostal vein
sv: subclavian vein
tent plex: tentorial plexus
vert v: vertebral vein

* unpaired midline structures

Figure 76. Infant
(153, 154, 149)
The internal jugular vein and its
tributaries

fv: facial vein
gcv: great cerebral vein
inf sag s: inferior sagittal
   sinus
ips: inferior petrosal sinus
os: occipital sinus
rbc: right brachiocephalic vein
scv: superior cerebral veins
si: left superior intercostal
   vein
sov: superior ophthalmic vein
sps: superior petrosal sinus
sv: subclavian vein

* unpaired midline structures

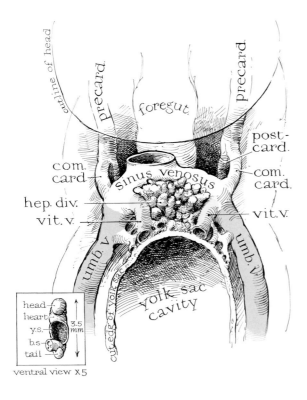

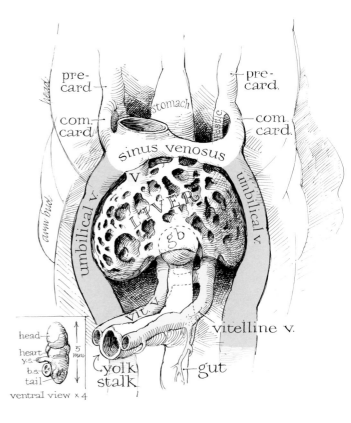

Figure 77. Stage 12
3–5 mm   26 days
21–29 pairs of somites
(32, 60, 149, 153, 154)
The liver and the umbilical veins

bs: body stalk
com card: common cardinal vein
hep div: hepatic diverticulum
postcard: postcardinal vein
precard: precardinal vein
umb v: umbilical vein
vit v: vitelline vein
ys: yolk sac

Figure 78. Stage 13
4–6 mm   28 days
30 or more pairs of somites
(61, 146, 149, 153, 154)
The liver and umbilical veins

bs: body stalk
com card: common cardinal vein
gb: gallbladder
post c: postcardinal vein
precard: precardinal vein
v: right hepatocardiac channel
vit v: vitelline vein
ys: yolk stalk

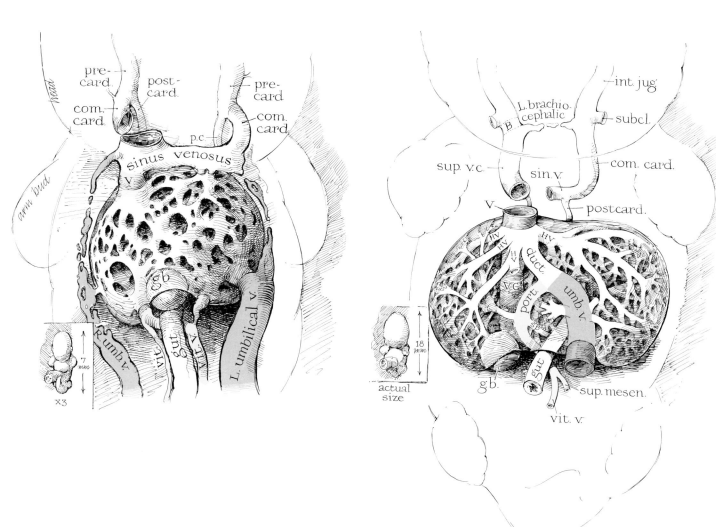

Figure 79. Stage 14
5–7 mm   32 days
(61, 86, 146, 149)
The liver and umbilical veins

com card: common cardinal vein
gb: gallbladder
precard: precardinal vein
pc: postcardinal vein
R umb v: right umbilical vein
v: right hepatocardiac channel
vit: right vitelline vein
vit v: left vitelline vein

Figure 80. Stage 19
16–18 mm   48 days
(63, 66, 149, 153, 154)
The liver and the umbilical vein

B: right brachiocephalic vein
com card: right common cardinal vein
gb: gallbladder
HV: hepatic vein
int jug: internal jugular vein
port: portal vein
postcard: postcardinal vein
sin v: sinus venosus
sp: splenic vein
subcl: subclavian vein
sup vc: superior vena cava
V: right hepatocardiac channel
VC: inferior vena cava
vit v: vitelline vein

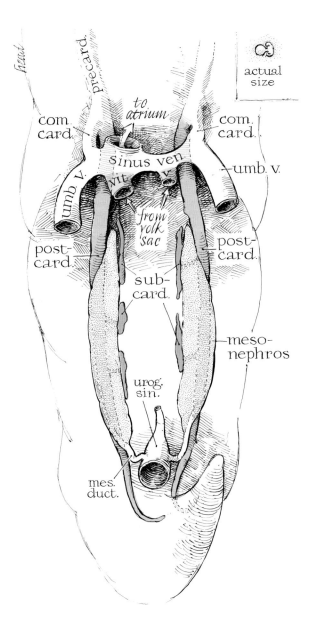

Figure 81. Stage 12
3–5 mm   26 days
21–29 pairs of somites
(147, 148, 150, 151)
The postcardinal and subcardinal veins

com card: common cardinal vein
mes duct: mesonephric duct

precard: precardinal vein
postcard: postcardinal vein
subcard: subcardinal vein
umb v: umbilical vein
urog sin: urogenital sinus
v: left vitelline vein
vit: right vitelline vein

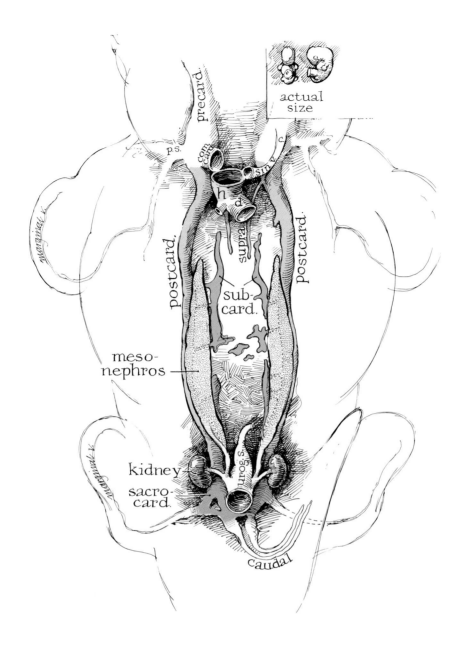

Figure 82. Stage 16
8–11 mm   37 days
(62, 148, 150, 151, 153, 154)
The postcardinal and subcardinal veins

d: ductus venosus
c: left common cardinal vein
com card: right common cardinal vein
h: right hepatocardiac channel

ps: primitive subclavian vein
postcard: postcardinal vein
precard: precardinal vein
sacrocard: sacrocardinal vein
sin v: sinus venosus
subcard: subcardinal veins
supra: supracardinal veins
urog sin: urogenital sinus

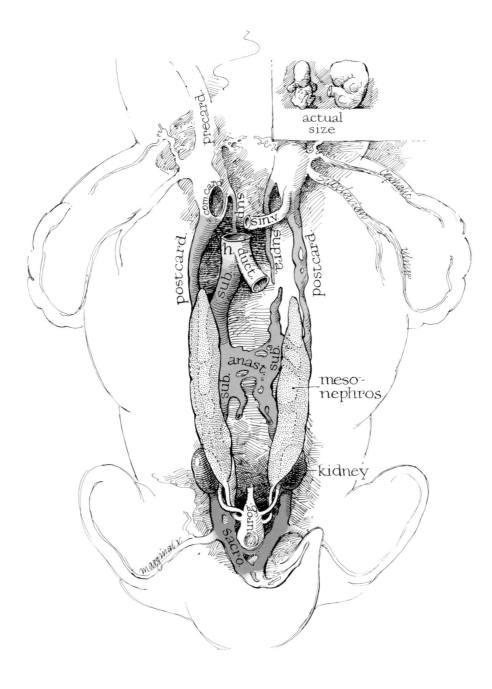

Figure 83. Stage 17
11–14 mm   41 days
(62, 148, 150, 151, 153, 154)
The postcardinal and subcardinal veins

anast: anastomosis between right and left
   subcardinal veins
com card: right common cardinal vein
duct: ductus venosus

h: right hepatocardiac channel
postcard: postcardinal vein
precard: precardinal vein
sacro: sacrocardinal vein
sin v: sinus venosus
sub: subcardinal vein
sup; supra: right and left supracardinal
   veins
urog sin: urogenital sinus

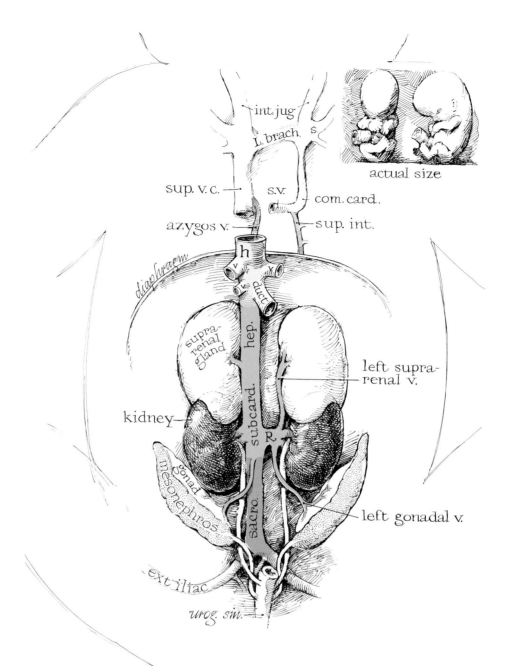

Figure 84. Stage 22
23–28 mm   54 days
(63, 148, 150, 151, 153, 154)
The inferior vena cava

duct: ductus venosus

h: suprahepatic part of inferior vena cava, derived from right hepatocardiac channel

hep: hepatic part of inferior vena cava, derived from anastomosis of right hepatocardiac channel and right subcardinal vein

L brach: left brachiocephalic vein

sv: sinus venosus (future coronary sinus)

sacro: sacrocardinal part of inferior vena

cava, derived from right sacrocardinal vein

subcard: subcardinal part of inferior vena cava, derived from right subcardinal vein

sup int: proximal part of left superior intercostal vein, derived from left postcardinal vein

sup vc: superior vena cava, derived from right common cardinal vein and proximal part of right precardinal vein

R: left renal vein, derived from anastomosis of right and left subcardinal veins

v: hepatic veins

Table 6. The Veins (148, 151)

Embryonic structure	Adult structure
Right vitelline vein	Contributes to portal vein; proximal part persists as right hepatocardiac channel (inferior vena cava from liver to heart).
Left vitelline vein	Forms most of portal vein
Ductus venosus	Ligamentum venosum
Left umbilical vein	Round ligament of liver
Right and left precardinal veins	Internal jugular veins
Right precardinal vein	Right brachiocephalic vein; contributes to superior vena cava
Right common cardinal vein	Contributes to superior vena cava
Left common cardinal vein	Lateral part of coronary sinus; oblique vein of left atrium
Right postcardinal vein	Proximal part of azygos vein
Left postcardinal vein	Left superior intercostal vein
Right subcardinal vein	Right gonadal vein; contributes to inferior vena cava
Left subcardinal vein	Left suprarenal vein; left gonadal vein; contributes to left renal vein
Supracardinal veins	Hemiazygos vein; caudal part of azygos vein
Right sacrocardinal vein	Right common iliac vein; contributes to inferior vena cava
Left sacrocardinal vein	Left common iliac vein
Caudal veins	Median sacral vein

The Nervous System

THE SPINAL CORD

The portion of the neural tube caudal to the fifth pair of somites becomes the spinal cord. During the fourth week a longitudinal groove termed the *sulcus limitans* develops along the inner wall of the central canal. The neural tube dorsal to the sulcus limitans on each side is termed the *alar plate,* and the neural tube ventral to the sulcus limitans on each side is termed the *basal plate.* The right and left alar plates are connected in the midline by a layer of ependymal and neuroglial cells termed the *roof plate;* the right and left basal plates are connected by a similar layer termed the *floor plate.*

By the middle of the fifth week three concentric layers can be distinguished in the spinal cord: an inner *ependymal layer,* a middle *mantle layer,* and an outer *marginal layer.*

The ependymal layer forms the epithelium which lines the central canal of the spinal cord and the ventricles of the brain. It also forms the epithelial components of the choroid plexuses.

The mantle layer consists primarily of cell bodies of neuroblasts, which form the gray matter of the central nervous system. The mantle layer of the alar plate forms the dorsal horn of the spinal cord. The mantle layer of the basal plate forms the ventral and lateral horns of the spinal cord.

The marginal layer becomes the white matter of the central nervous system. It consists of a framework of supporting cells into which processes of nerve cells grow to form the spinal tracts.

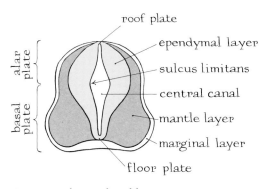

Stage 17 6th week (166)
Transverse section through the upper thoracic region of the spinal cord

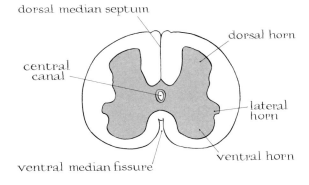

12th week (170)
Transverse section through the cervical region of the spinal cord

During the latter part of the embryonic period the spinal cord extends well into the coccygeal region. During the fetal period, however, the coccygeal portion of the cord regresses and forms the filum terminale. At the same time, the vertebral column grows more rapidly than the spinal cord, with the result that at birth the lower end of the spinal cord lies at the level of the third lumbar vertebra. This process continues into childhood until the caudal end of the spinal cord reaches its final position opposite the first lumbar vertebra.

THE BRAIN

The portion of the neural tube cranial to the fifth pair of somites becomes the brain. Early in embryonic development the primordium of the brain and the spinal cord resemble each other in many respects. The ependymal, mantle, and marginal layers can be identified in all divisions of the brain, as can the roof plate and the alar plates. The basal plates, however, are confined to the midbrain and the hindbrain, and the floorplate is found only in the hindbrain.

As in the spinal cord, the neuroblasts which originate in the alar plate of the embryonic brain are primarily sensory and associative in function, whereas the neuroblasts originating in the basal plate are primarily motor. This basic pattern is radically modified, however, by the invasion of fiber tracts and by the proliferation and migration of neuroblasts. For example, in the cerebrum and the cerebellum, neuroblasts migrate from the mantle layer into the marginal layer, where they form the cerebral and cerebellar cortices. The remaining cells of the mantle layer form masses of gray matter termed *nuclei*.

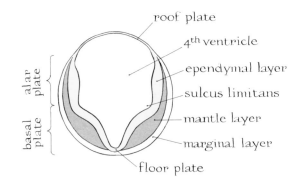

Stage 17   6th week (170)
Transverse section through the myelencephalon

Primary divisions of the brain

While the neural tube is closing, the three primary divisions of the brain develop as local enlargements at the cranial end of the neural tube. These divisions are the *hindbrain,* or *rhombencephalon;* the *midbrain,* or *mesencephalon;* and the *forebrain,* or *prosencephalon.* Subsequently the rhombencephalon gives rise to two secondary divisions: the *myelencephalon* and the *metencephalon.* The prosencephalon gives rise to the *diencephalon* and the *telencephalon.*

The flexures

During the fourth week the rapid growth of the brain results in the formation of two prominent flexures: the *cervical flexure,* between the hindbrain (rhombencephalon) and the spinal cord, and the *cephalic flexure,* in the region of the midbrain (mesencephalon). During the fifth week a third flexure, the *pontine flexure,* develops at the junction of the metencephalon and the myelencephalon.

Ventricles of the brain

The lumen of the neural tube becomes the central canal of the spinal cord and the ventricles of the brain. As the primary divisions of the brain undergo differentiation, the cavities corresponding to each division assume their final form.

The central canal of the spinal cord communicates with the *fourth ventricle,* which develops from the cavity of the hindbrain (rhombencephalon). The fourth ventricle is continuous with the *cerebral aqueduct,* or cavity of the midbrain (mesencephalon). The cerebral aqueduct opens into the *third ventricle,* which develops from the cavity of the diencephalon. The third ventricle communicates with the paired *lateral ventricles,* which are the cavities of the cerebral hemispheres.

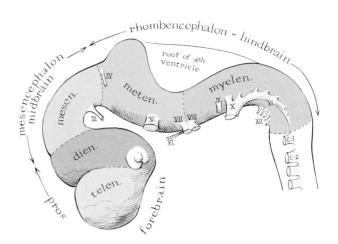

Stage 16   6th week (143)
The primary divisions of the brain

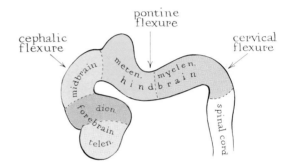

6th week (143)
The flexures as seen in the sixth week

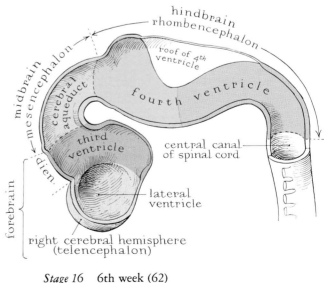

Stage 16   6th week (62)
Sagittal section of the brain

The myelencephalon

The myelencephalon (medulla oblongata) is the most caudal and in many ways the most primitive part of the brain. The basic structural pattern of the spinal cord is continued into the posterior end of the myelencephalon, but toward the anterior end it becomes more highly specialized as the primitive pattern is modified and new structures are added.

The cavity of the myelencephalon expands to form the posterior part of the fourth ventricle. At the same time, the ependymal tissue of the roof plate becomes greatly attenuated and fuses with the overlying *pia mater,* forming the posterior part of the roof of the fourth ventricle. Capillaries in the pia mater invaginate the ependyma to form the choroid plexus of the fourth ventricle.

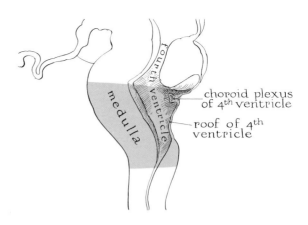

3d month (159)
Sagittal section of the myelencephalon

The metencephalon

At first the metencephalon resembles the myelencephalon, but in the course of its development it undergoes radical transformations. The roof plate becomes the medullary velum, which contributes to the roof of the fourth ventricle. The dorsolateral portions of the alar plates are modified to form the cerebellum, and the ventromedial portions of the alar plates contribute to the formation of the cerebral peduncles. The basal plate forms the pons.

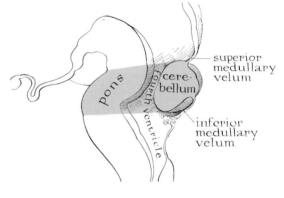

3d month (159)
Sagittal section of the metencephalon

The mesencephalon

The roof plate of the mesencephalon retains its identity until the second month, when it is absorbed into the alar plates as they form the tectum. The tectum consists of four rounded elevations termed the *corpora quadrigemina* or *superior* and *inferior colliculi.* The basal plates form the cerebral peduncles. They consist of a dorsal part, termed the *tegmentum,* and a ventral part, termed the *crus cerebri.*

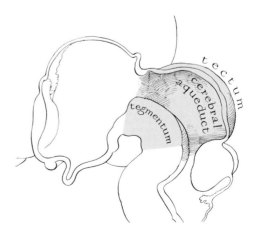

3d month (159)
Sagittal section of the mesencephalon

The diencephalon

The roof plate of the diencephalon is a thin ependymal layer which combines with vessels of the pia mater to form the choroid plexus of the third ventricle. During the seventh week the caudal part of the roof plate evaginates to form the pineal body (part of the epithalamus). The remainder of the epithalamus, as well as the thalamus and the hypothalamus, develops from the alar plates. The optic stalk is an outgrowth of the wall of the diencephalon, and the optic chiasma is considered part of the hypothalamus. Also included in the hypothalamus is the infundibular process, a ventral diverticulum which forms the neural lobe of the hypophysis.

The telencephalon

The cerebral hemispheres originate during the fifth week as paired evaginations from the anterior part of the lateral walls of the prosencephalon. They are considered derivatives of the alar plate.

Each cerebral hemisphere may be divided into two parts: the *pallium* and the *basal ganglia.* The pallium includes the cerebral cortex and the subjacent white matter. Certain neuroblasts of the mantle layer migrate into the marginal layer where they develop into the cerebral cortex; other neuroblasts of the mantle layer form the basal ganglia. The white matter of the pallium is derived from the marginal layer of the neural tube.

Each cerebral hemisphere contains a lateral ventricle which communicates with the third ventricle via an opening termed the *interventricular foramen.* As the lateral ventricles grow, choroid plexuses develop within them. These plexuses are similar in origin to the choroid plexuses of the third and fourth ventricles, and extend from the interventricular formaina into the anterior ends of the inferior horns of the lateral ventricles.

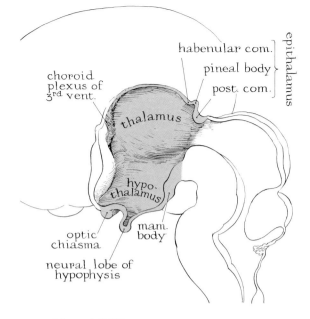

3d month (159)
Sagittal section of the diencephalon

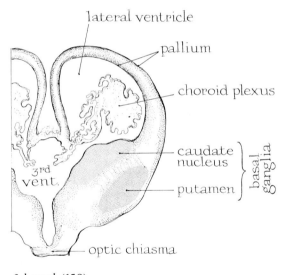

3d month (159)
Coronal section of the telencephalon

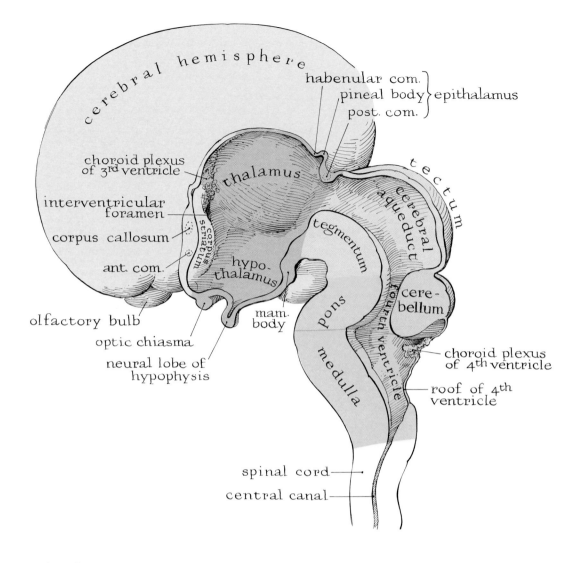

cerebral hemisphere

habenular com.
pineal body } epithalamus
post. com.

choroid plexus
of 3rd ventricle

thalamus

tectum

cerebral aqueduct

interventricular
foramen

corpus striatum

corpus callosum

tegmentum

cerebellum

ant. com.

hypo-
thalamus

pons

fourth ventricle

olfactory bulb

mam.
body

medulla

optic chiasma

neural lobe of
hypophysis

choroid plexus
of 4th ventricle

roof of 4th
ventricle

spinal cord

central canal

3d month (159)
Sagittal section of the brain

Table 7. Primary Divisions of the Brain

Prosencephalon = forebrain	Telencephalon	Cavity	Lateral (first and second) ventricles	
		Roof plate	Choroid plexus	
		Alar plate	Cerebral hemispheres	
	Diencephelon	Cavity	Third ventricle	
		Roof plate	Choroid plexus, pineal body	
		Alar plate	Epithalamus, thalamus, hypothalamus	
Mesencephalon = midbrain	Mesencephalon	Cavity	Cerebral aqueduct	
		Roof plate	Contributes to tectum	
		Alar plate	Tectum = corpora quadrigemina	Superior colliculus
				Inferior colliculus
		Basal plate	Cerebral peduncles	Tegmentum, motor nuclei III and IV
				crus cerebri
Rhombencephalon = hindbrain	Metencephalon	Cavity	Fourth ventricle (anterior part)	
		Roof plate	Medullary velum	
		Alar plate	Cerebellum; contributes to cerebral peduncles	
		Basal plate	Pons	Tegmentum, motor nuclei, V, VI, VII
				Basilar part
		Floor plate	Midline raphé	
	Myelencephalon = medulla oblongata	Cavity	Fourth ventricle (posterior part)	
		Roof plate	Ependyma + pia mater = roof of fourth ventricle and choroid plexus	
		Alar plate	Sensory relay nuclei VII, IX, X	
		Basal plate	Motor nuclei IX, X, XI, XII	
		Floor plate	Midline raphé	

Wilhelm His and other early embryologists made many attempts to draw parallels between the structure of the spinal cord and that of the brain. His believed that he could identify in the midbrain and forebrain structures homologous to all the components of the spinal cord, but his findings were not universally accepted. The subject was reviewed in three classic papers by B. F. Kingsbury (160, 161, 162), and it is Kingsbury's account which is followed here.

THE SPINAL NERVES

The spinal nerves originate from two sources: *motor neuroblasts* in the basal plate, and *sensory neuroblasts* derived from the neural crest.

1. Each motor neuroblast gives rise to a process termed the *primitive axon*, which emerges from the ventrolateral wall of the spinal cord and grows distally to enter a skeletal muscle. At the same time, primitive dendrites appear on the side of the cell body opposite the axon.

2. The primordia of the spinal ganglia consist primarily of sensory neuroblasts. Each sensory neuroblast gives rise to two processes: one process grows distally and terminates in a sensory receptor or as a free nerve ending; the other process grows toward the spinal cord and penetrates the dorsal horn.

The axons which arise from motor neuroblasts in the basal plate collectively form the ventral, or motor roots of the spinal nerves. The processes which arise from sensory neuroblasts in the spinal ganglia collectively form the dorsal, or sensory roots of the spinal nerves.

Distal to the spinal ganglion the dorsal and ventral roots unite to form the spinal nerve. By the end of the fifth week the principal branches of each spinal nerve can be identified. They are:

1. *The dorsal primary division.* The dorsal primary divisions of the spinal nerves supply the muscles and the skin of the dorsal part of the neck and trunk.

2. *The ventral primary division.* The ventral primary divisions of the spinal nerves supply the muscles and skin of the ventral and lateral parts of the trunk and all parts of the arms and the legs.

3. *The rami communicantes.* The rami communicantes consist of visceral afferent and autonomic fibers which connect the spinal nerves to the sympathetic ganglia. The autonomic components of the spinal nerves are described on page 118.

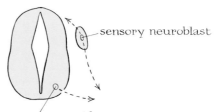

Stage 13   4 weeks
Transverse section through the spinal cord (schematic). Dotted lines indicate direction of growth of neuroblast processes.

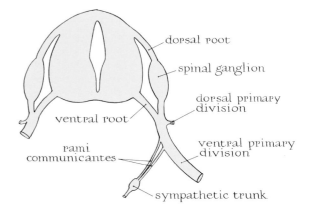

Stage 19   7 weeks
Transverse section through the spinal cord

THE CRANIAL NERVES

Branchial arch nerves

Certain structural features of spinal nerves can be identified in cranial nerves. Cranial nerves V (trigeminal), VII (facial), IX (glossopharyngeal), X (vagus), and XI (accessory) bear the greatest resemblance to spinal nerves. They are termed *branchial arch nerves* because they innervate muscles which have evolved from the branchial (gill) arch musculature of primitive fishes. They resemble the spinal nerves in that they include sensory fibers which originate from neural crest cells outside the neural tube, and motor fibers which originate from neuroblasts in the basal plate of the neural tube. In other respects, however, they are highly specialized and cannot be considered serial homologs of spinal nerves.

Somatic motor nerves

Cranial nerves III (oculomotor), IV (trochlear), and VI (abducent) innervate the eye muscles. Cranial nerve XII (hypoglossal) innervates the muscles of the tongue. Phylogenetically, the muscles of the eye and the tongue are derived from somites and these nerves are therefore termed *somatic motor nerves.* They resemble the ventral roots of spinal nerves in that they consist for the most part of somatic motor fibers which originate from neuroblasts in the basal plate of the neural tube.

Unlike the branchial arch nerves, the somatic motor nerves do not have sensory ganglia which lie outside the brain. Nerves III, IV, and VI do contain proprioceptive fibers, but these fibers arise from cell bodies within the brain stem, and thus constitute an exception to the rule that primary sensory neurons are situated in peripheral ganglia.

Special sensory nerves

Cranial nerves I (olfactory), II (optic), and VIII (acoustic) are termed *special sensory nerves.* They are highly specialized and bear little or no resemblance to spinal nerves.

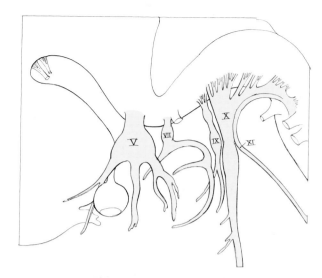

Stage 19   7th week (143)
The branchial arch nerves

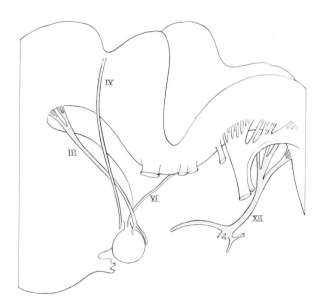

Stage 19   7th week (143)
The somatic motor nerves

The autonomic system

The autonomic system differs from the somatic motor system both in structure and function. Functionally the autonomic system is distinguished by the fact that it conveys motor impulses to smooth muscle, cardiac muscle, and glands, whereas the somatic motor system conveys impulses to the skeletal (striated) muscles. Structurally, the two systems differ in the number of neurons required to transmit an impulse from the central nervous system to an effector organ. Only one neuron is required to transmit somatic motor impulses, but autonomic impulses are transmitted by a chain of at least two neurons. The cell body of the first neuron is located within the central nervous system, and the cell body of the second neuron is located in one of the peripheral autonomic ganglia outside the central nervous system.

These two neurons have different embryonic origins. The neurons with cell bodies in peripheral autonomic ganglia originate from the neural crest. Early in the fifth week certain neural crest cells migrate ventrally and begin aggregating to form the sympathetic trunk and other ganglia and plexuses of the autonomic system. Later in the same week, axons arising from autonomic neuroblasts in the mantle layer of the neural tube grow toward the ganglia and begin to establish synaptic contact with the cells of neural crest origin.

The autonomic system can be divided into two components, termed the *sympathetic* and *parasympathetic systems*. The embryonic origins of these two systems are listed in Table 8, on the facing page.

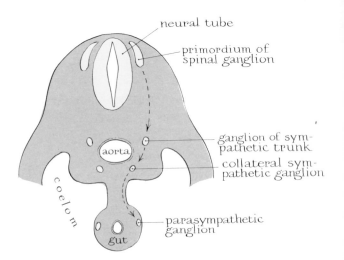

Stage 15 5th week
Transverse section through the abdominal region in the fifth week (schematic). Dotted lines indicate the path of migrating neural crest cells.

Table 8. Functional Components of Cerebral and Spinal Nerves and Their Embryonic Origins (9, 11)

		Embryonic origin of neuroblast	Location of cell bodies in adult	Peripheral distribution of fibers
Somatic	Somatic afferent (sensory) Conscious sensation: pain, temperature, touch, and proprioceptive sensation from muscles and joints	Neural crest	Sensory ganglia of cerebral and spinal nerves	All spinal nerves Certain cranial nerves
	Somatic efferent (motor) Voluntary movements: motor impulses to muscles	Basal plate of neural tube	Ventral horn of spinal cord Ventral part of brain stem	All spinal nerves Certain cranial nerves
Visceral	Visceral afferent (sensory) Vaguely localised and subconscious sensations from viscera	Neural crest	Sensory ganglia of cerebral and spinal nerves	All spinal nerves Certain cranial nerves Sympathetic trunk Splanchnic nerves Autonomic plexuses
	Visceral efferent (motor) or Autonomic system Motor impulses to viscera Largely involuntary	Neural crest and Basal plate of neural tube	Peripheral autonomic ganglia Lateral horn of spinal cord Ventral part of brain stem	All spinal nerves Certain cranial nerves Autonomic nerves, plexuses, and ganglia

Table 9. Embryonic Origin of the Autonomic System (9, 11)

		Embryonic origin of neuroblast	Location of cell bodies in adult	Peripheral distribution of fibers
Visceral efferent (motor) or autonomic system	Sympathetic	Neural crest	Ganglia of sympathetic trunk and collateral sympathetic ganglia	Gray rami communicantes, sympathetic chain and its branches
		Basal plate of neural tube (thoracic and upper lumbar segments)	Lateral horn of spinal cord (T-1 to T-12 and L-1 to L-2)	White rami communicantes, splanchnic nerves, etc.
	Parasympathetic	Neural crest	Peripheral ganglia near organs innervated	Fibers from ganglia to viscera
		Basal plate of neural tube (brain stem and sacral region)	Brain stem, lateral horn of spinal cord S-2, 3, 4	Cranial nerves III, VII, IX, X, and pelvic splanchnic nerves

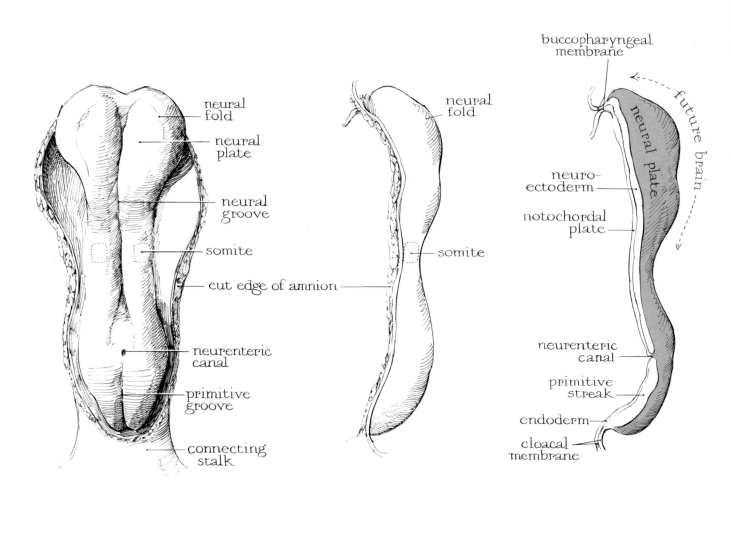

dorsal view | lateral view | sagittal section

Figure 85. Stage 9
1 somite
(45, **49**, 57, 82)
The development of the neural tube

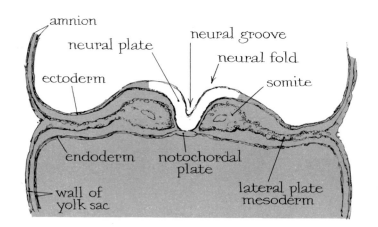

transverse section

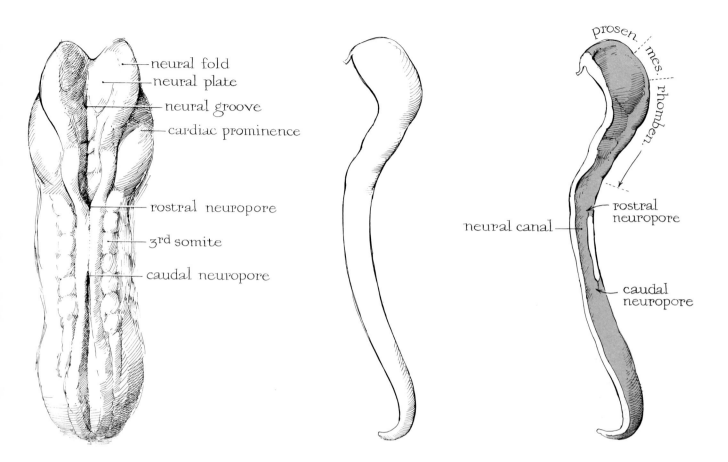

dorsal view of embryo   lateral view of neural tube   sagittal section of neural tube

Figure 86. Stage 10
7 somites
(31, **51**, 54, 64, 70, 75, 164)
The development of the neural tube

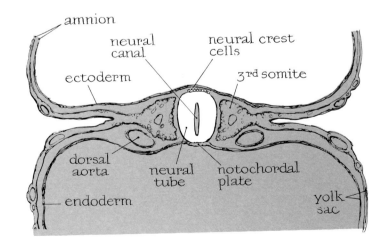

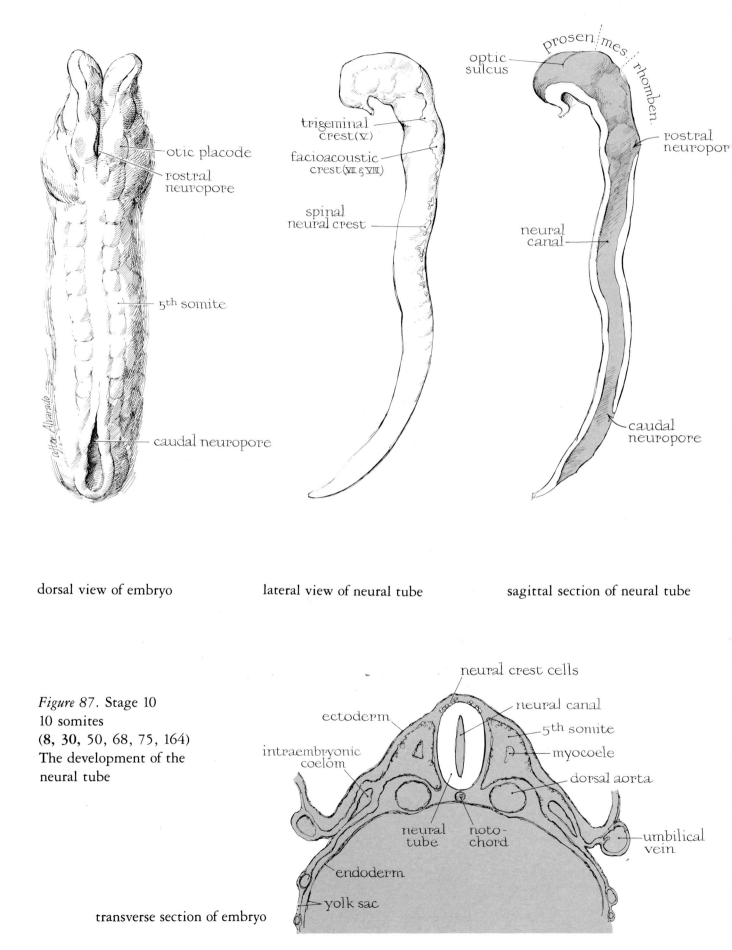

otic placode

rostral
neuropore

5th somite

caudal neuropore

dorsal view of embryo

trigeminal
crest (V)

facioacoustic
crest (VII & VIII)

spinal
neural crest

lateral view of neural tube

optic
sulcus

prosen. / mes. / rhomben.

rostral
neuropor

neural
canal

caudal
neuropore

sagittal section of neural tube

Figure 87. Stage 10
10 somites
(**8, 30, 50, 68, 75, 164**)
The development of the
neural tube

neural crest cells

ectoderm

neural canal

5th somite

myocoele

intraembryonic
coelom

dorsal aorta

neural
tube

noto-
chord

umbilical
vein

endoderm

yolk sac

transverse section of embryo

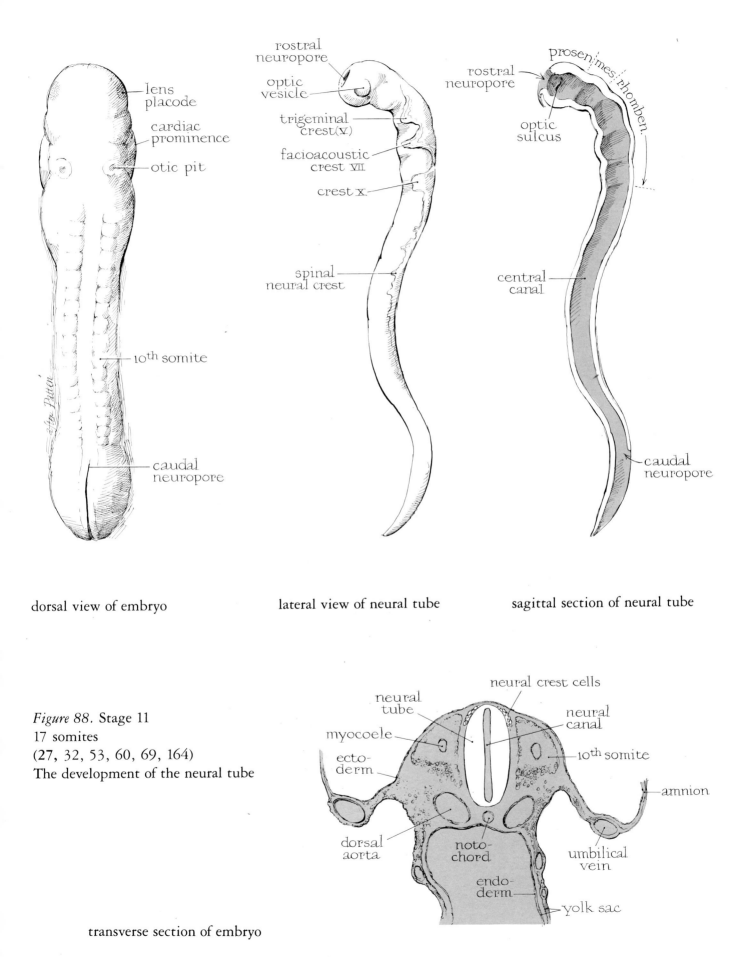

dorsal view of embryo

lateral view of neural tube

sagittal section of neural tube

Figure 88. Stage 11
17 somites
(**27**, 32, 53, 60, 69, 164)
The development of the neural tube

transverse section of embryo

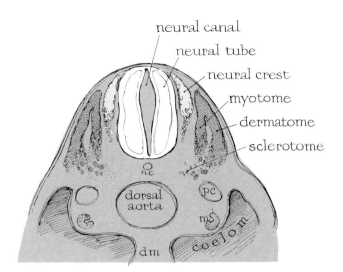

neural canal
neural tube
neural crest
myotome
dermatome
sclerotome

dorsal aorta
pc
n.c.
m
coelom
dm

Figure 89. Stage 13
4–6 mm   28 days
30 or more pairs of somites
(43, 166, 220)
Transverse section through
the spinal cord and adjacent
structures

dm: dorsal mesentery
m: mesonephros
nc: notochord
pc: postcardinal vein

Figure 90. Stage 13 (facing page)
4–6 mm   28 days
30 or more pairs of somites
(43, 143, 156, 159)
Lateral view of the neural tube

C-1: first cervical neural crest
T-1: first thoracic neural crest
L-1: first lumbar neural crest

Cranial nerves:
    V: trigeminal ganglion
        V-1: ophthalmic nerve
        V-2: maxillary nerve
        V-3: mandibular nerve
    VII: facial nerve
    VIII: vestibulocochlear nerve
    IX: glossopharyngeal nerve
    X: vagus nerve
    XI: accessory nerve
    XII: hypoglossal nerve

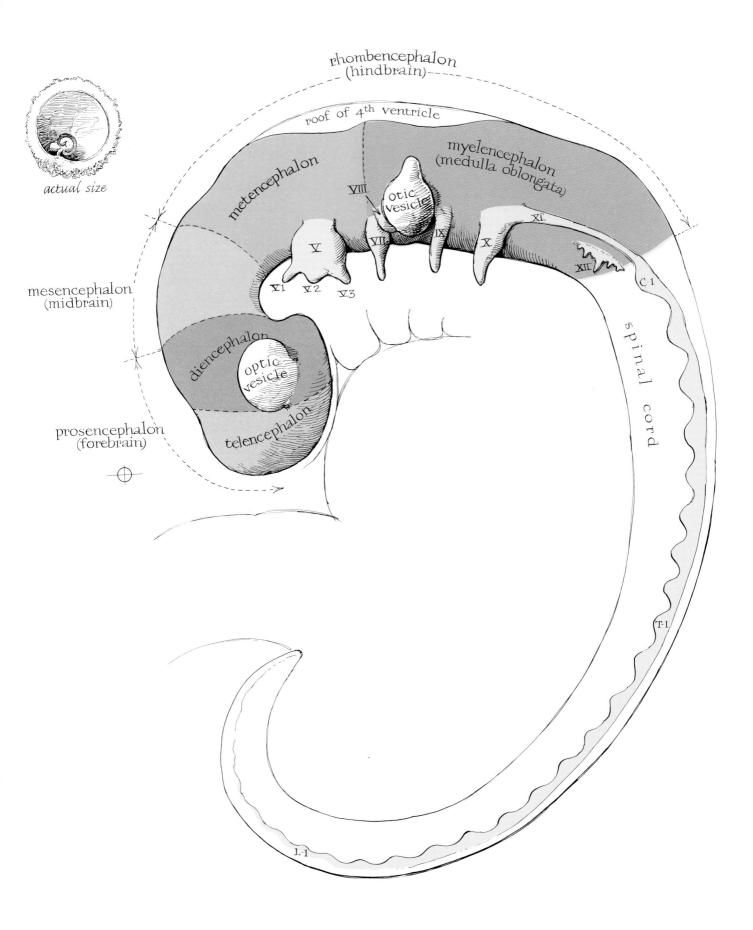

rhombencephalon
(hindbrain)

roof of 4th ventricle

metencephalon

myelencephalon
(medulla oblongata)

VIII

otic
vesicle

V

VII

IX

X

XI

V1   V2   V3

XII

C-1

mesencephalon
(midbrain)

diencephalon

optic
vesicle

spinal cord

prosencephalon
(forebrain)

telencephalon

actual size

T-1

L-1

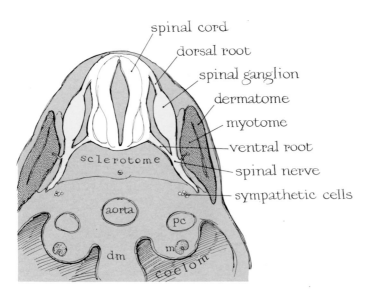

spinal cord
dorsal root
spinal ganglion
dermatome
myotome
ventral root
spinal nerve
sympathetic cells
sclerotome
aorta
pc
dm
m
coelom

Figure 91. Stage 14
5–7 mm   32 days
(220, 33, 52, 167)
Transverse section through
the spinal cord and adjacent
structures

dm: dorsal mesentery
m: mesonephros
pc: postcardinal vein

Figure 92. Stage 14 (facing page)
5–7 mm   32 days
(33, 52, 61, 143, 159, 168)
Lateral view of the nervous system

trig gang: trigeminal ganglion

Cranial nerves:
   C-1: spinal ganglion of first cervical nerve
   T-1: spinal ganglion of first thoracic nerve
   L-1: spinal ganglion of first lumbar nerve
   III: oculomotor nerve
   IV: trochlear nerve
   V: trigeminal nerve
      V-1: ophthalmic nerve
      V-2: maxillary nerve
      V-3: mandibular nerve
   VII: facial nerve
   VIII: vestibulocochlear nerve
   IX: glossopharyngeal nerve
   X: vagus nerve
   XI: accessory nerve
   XII: hypoglossal nerve

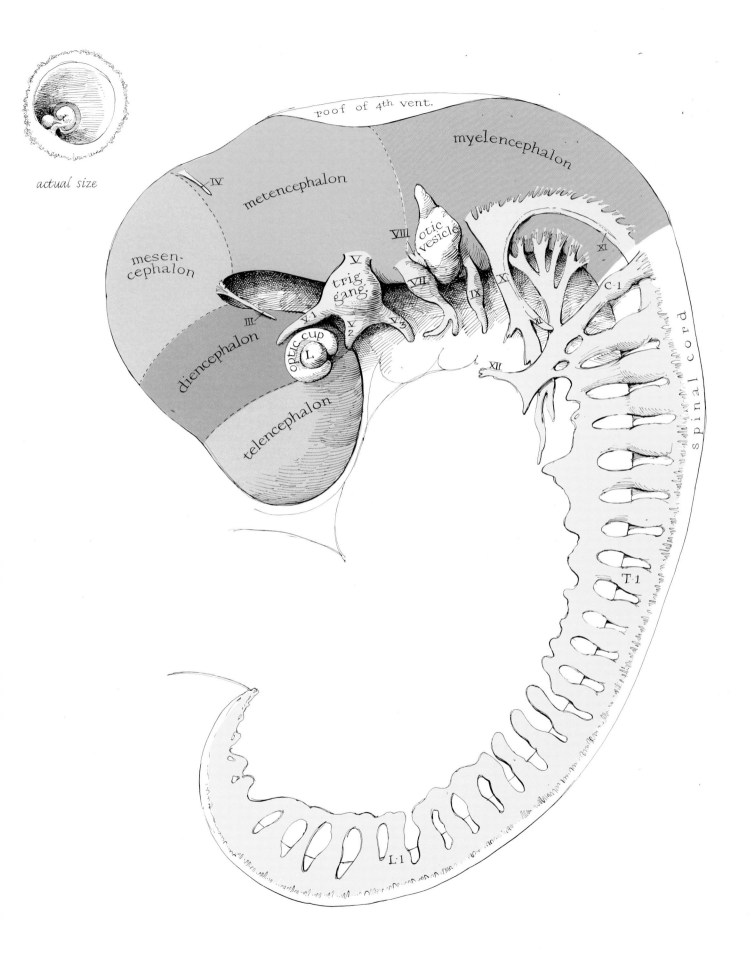

actual size

roof of 4th vent.

myelencephalon

metencephalon

IV

mesen-
cephalon

VIII

otic
vesicle

XI

V

trig.
gang.

VII

X

C·1

III

V 1

IX

XI

optic cup

L.

V 2

V 3

XII

diencephalon

telencephalon

spinal cord

T·1

L·1

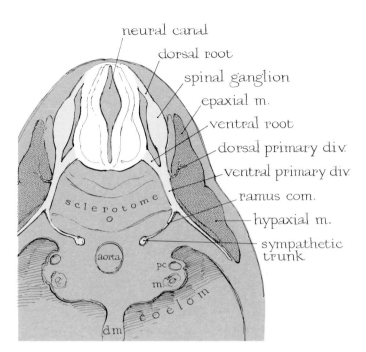

neural canal
dorsal root
spinal ganglion
epaxial m.
ventral root
dorsal primary div.
ventral primary div.
ramus com.
hypaxial m.
sympathetic trunk
sclerotome
aorta
pc
m
coelom
dm

Figure 93. Stage 16
8–11 mm   37 days
(220)
Transverse section through
the spinal cord and adjacent
structures

dm: dorsal mesentery
m: mesonephros
pc: postcardinal vein

Figure 94. Stage 16 (facing page)
8–11 mm   37 days
(143, 159, 168, 169, 220, 221, 223, 224)
Lateral view of the nervous system

ac: ansa cervicalis
C-1: spinal ganglion of first cervical nerve
cp: common peroneal nerve
fe: femoral nerve
L: lens
L-1: spinal ganglion of first lumbar nerve
me: median nerve
mem lab: membranous labyrinth
ph: phrenic nerve
ob: obturator nerve
ra: radial nerve
sc: sciatic nerve
S-1: spinal ganglion of first sacral nerve
T-1: spinal ganglion of first thoracic nerve
trig gang: trigeminal ganglion
ul: ulnar nerve

Cranial nerves:
   III: oculomotor nerve
   IV: trochlear nerve
   V: trigeminal nerve
      V-1: ophthalmic nerve
      V-2: maxillary nerve
      V-3: mandibular nerve
   VI: abducent nerve
   VII: facial nerve
   VIII: vestibulocochlear nerve
   IX: glossopharyngeal nerve
   X: vagus nerve
   XI: accessory nerve
   XII: hypoglossal nerve

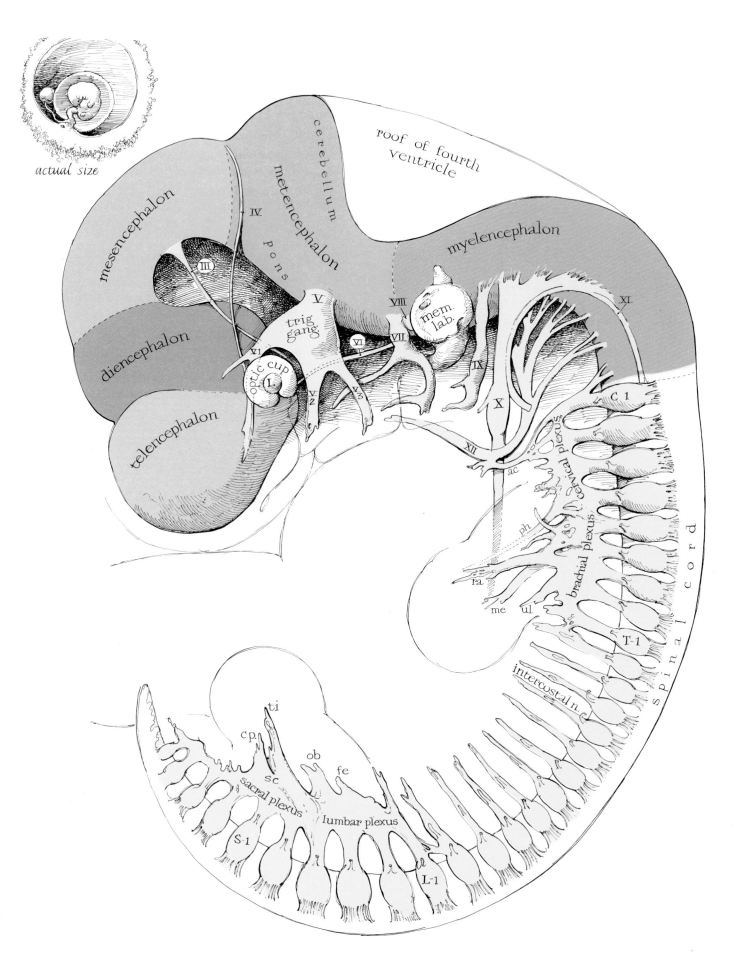

actual size

mesencephalon

cerebellum

metencephalon

roof of fourth
ventricle

IV

pons

myelencephalon

III

diencephalon

V

trig.
gang.

VIII

mem.
lab.

XI

VI

VII

optic cup

v1

IX

telencephalon

v2

X

v3

XII

C 1

ac

cervical plexus

ph

brachial plexus

spinal cord

ra

me   ul

T-1

intercostal n.

ti

cp.

ob

fe

sc

S-1

sacral plexus

lumbar plexus

L-1

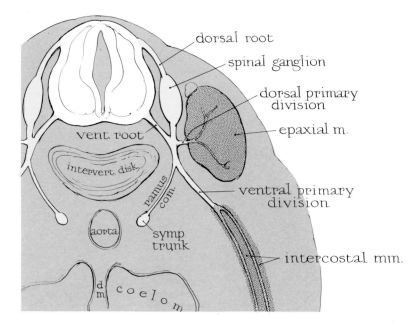

dorsal root
spinal ganglion
dorsal primary division
epaxial m.
vent. root
intervert. disk
ramus com.
ventral primary division
aorta
symp trunk
intercostal mm.
d m coelom

Figure 95. Stage 19
16–18 mm   47 days
(170)
Transverse section through
the spinal cord and adjacent
structures

Figure 96. Stage 19 (facing page)
16–18 mm   47 days
(156, 168, 220, 221, 224)
Lateral view of the nervous system

ac: ansa cervicalis
C-1: spinal ganglion of first cervical nerve
cp: common peroneal nerve
fe: femoral nerve
L-1: spinal ganglion of first lumbar nerve
m: membranous labyrinth
me: median nerve
ph: phrenic nerve
ob: obturator nerve
ra: radial nerve
sc: sciatic nerve
S-1: spinal ganglion of first sacral nerve
T-1: spinal ganglion of first thoracic nerve
trig gang: trigeminal ganglion
ul: ulnar nerve

Cranial nerves:
   I: olfactory nerve
   III: oculomotor nerve
   IV: trochlear nerve
   V: trigeminal nerve
      V-1: ophthalmic nerve
      V-2: maxillary nerve
      V-3: mandibular nerve
   VI: abducent nerve
   VII: facial nerve
   VIII: vestibulocochlear nerve
   IX: glossopharyngeal nerve
   X: vagus nerve
   XI: accessory nerve
   XII: hypoglossal nerve

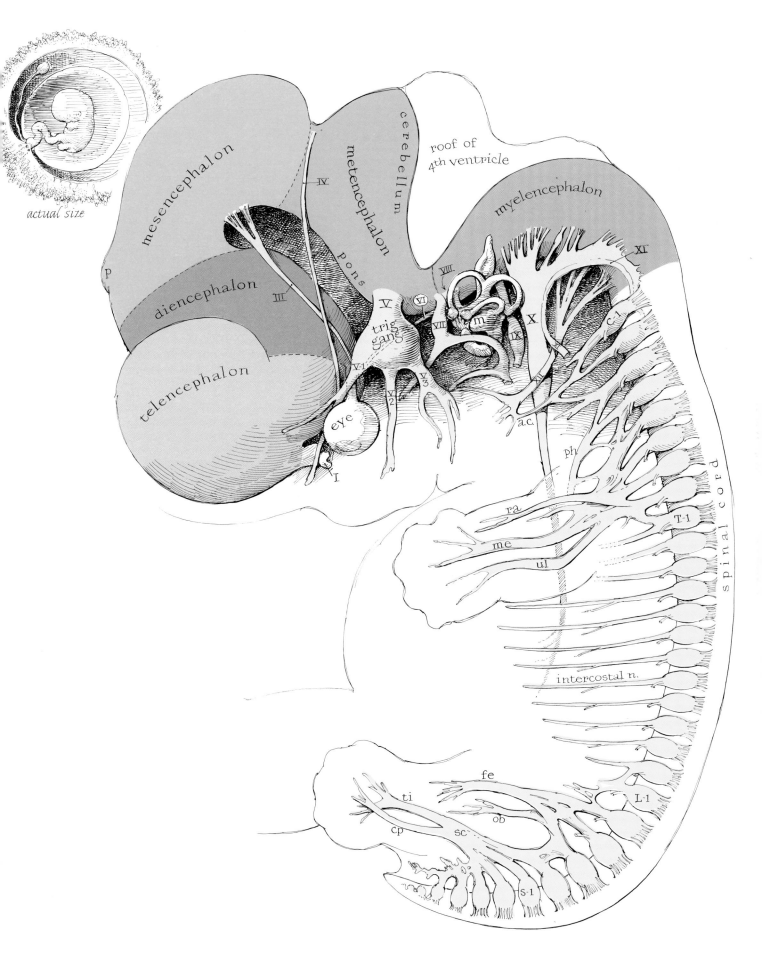

actual size

mesencephalon

cerebellum

metencephalon

roof of
4th ventricle

myelencephalon

pons

IV

P

diencephalon

III

XI

VIII

V

VI

telencephalon

trig
gang

VII

m

X

IX

C-1

V-1

XI

V-3

V-2

eye

a.c.

I

ph

ra

me

ul

T-1

spinal cord

intercostal n.

fe

ti

L-1

cp

ob

sc

S-1

The Eye

The optic vesicle

During the fourth week paired evaginations termed *optic vesicles* develop on either side of the prosencephalon (forebrain) and bulge into the adjacent mesenchyme. The cavity of each optic vesicle is continuous with the cavity of the prosencephalon, and each vesicle is attached to the prosencephalon by a short tubular *optic stalk.*

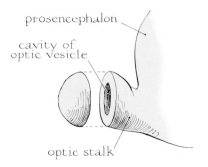

Stage 13   4 weeks (172)
Section of the optic vesicle

The optic cup and the retina

Toward the end of the fourth week the lateral wall of the optic vesicle invaginates, forming a concave, double-walled structure termed the *optic cup.* The invagination extends along the inferior surface of the optic stalk, with the result that the lower part of the cup and the stalk are marked by a groove termed the *optic fissure.* The outer layer of the optic cup becomes the pigmented layer of the retina, and the inner layer forms the nervous tissues of the retina. The space between the two layers is termed the *intraretinal space.* The rim of the optic cup *(pars caeca retina)* contributes to the formation of the ciliary body and the iris.

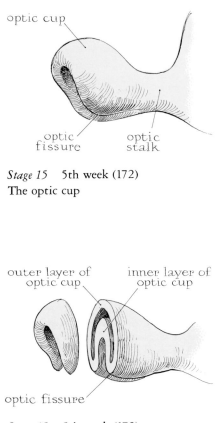

Stage 15   5th week (172)
The optic cup

Stage 15   5th week (172)
Section of optic cup

132

The lens

As the optic vesicle develops, its lateral wall approaches the overlying ectoderm, and at this point a thickened area of ectoderm termed the *lens placode* develops. When the optic vesicle invaginates the lens placode also invaginates, forming a *lens vesicle* which comes to lie within the optic cup. By the beginning of the sixth week the lens vesicle breaks free from the surface ectoderm. The growth of the lens continues throughout the fetal period and well into the postnatal period.

The sclera and the cornea

During the seventh week the brain and the optic cup are surrounded by a condensation of mesenchyme. The part around the brain forms the *dura mater,* and the part around the optic cup forms the *sclera* and the *stroma of the cornea.* The outer epithelial layer of the cornea is derived from ectoderm.

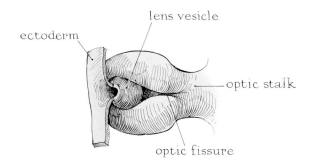
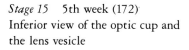

Stage 15   5th week (172)
Inferior view of the optic cup and the lens vesicle

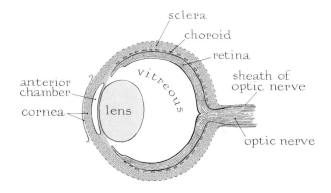

3d month (172)
Schematic section of the eye in third month

133

The choroid, the iris, and the ciliary body

The *choroid* is a vascular membrane which lies between the sclera and the retina. It originates from mesenchyme, and is an extension of the same primitive vascular coat which forms the cranial pia mater.

The *iris* is derived from two sources: neural ectoderm and mesenchyme.

Mesenchyme forms the *pupillary membrane.* This membrane originates during the eighth week as a result of the development of the anterior chamber. It covers the anterior surface of the lens until the latter part of the fetal period, when its central portion degenerates. The peripheral part of the pupillary membrane forms the stroma, or supporting connective tissue of the iris. The pigmented epithelium and the smooth muscles of the iris develop from the anterior portion of the rim of the optic cup.

The *ciliary body* lies between the iris and the neural part of the retina. The epithelial portion of the ciliary body is derived from the rim of the optic cup; the stroma and the ciliary muscle are derived from adjacent mesenchyme.

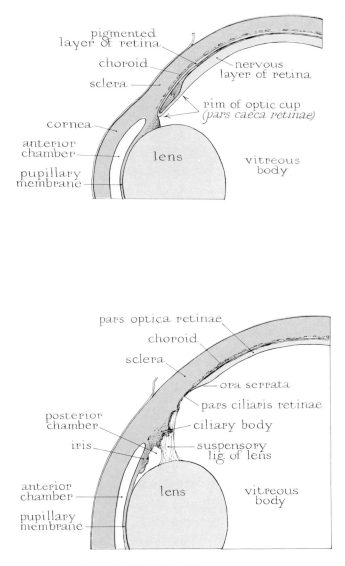

6 months (172, 173, 177)
Section of the anterior part of the eye

134

The anterior and posterior chambers and the vitreous body

During the eighth week the *anterior chamber* appears as a space in the mesenchyme between the lens and the cornea. Its posterior wall is formed by the pupillary membrane. Later in fetal development the forward growth of the iris results in the formation of a small space termed the *posterior chamber* between the lens and the iris. Initially the anterior and posterior chambers are separated by the pupillary membrane, but when the central portion of the pupillary membrane degenerates, the anterior and posterior chambers communicate with each other via the pupil. Both chambers are filled with a clear fluid termed the *aqueous humor.*

The space between the posterior surface of the lens and the retina is filled by a gelatinous substance termed the *vitreous body.* Its embryonic origin is not fully understood. It is thought to be derived from the inner layer of the optic cup, but mesenchyme which invades the optic cup via the optic fissure may also play a role in its development.

The optic nerve

During the seventh week the edges of the optic fissure meet and fuse around the hyaloid artery (see below) with the result that the artery becomes enclosed within the optic stalk. At the same time, nerve fibers originating from ganglion cells in the inner layer of the optic cup grow through the inner part of the optic stalk toward the brain and the cavity of the optic stalk becomes obliterated. These nerve fibers, together with supporting tissue derived from the outer portion of the optic stalk, constitute the optic nerve.

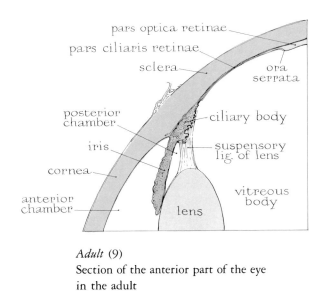

Adult (9)
Section of the anterior part of the eye in the adult

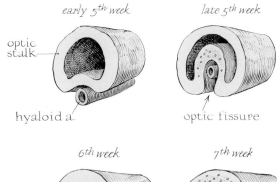

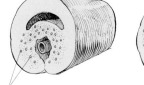

Early 5th-7th week (172, 177)
The transformation of the optic stalk and the development of optic nerve fibers

The hyaloid artery

The vitreous body and the lens are supplied by the *hyaloid artery,* a branch of the ophthalmic artery which enters the optic cup through the optic fissure. During the fetal period branches of the hyaloid artery spread out in the retina, and toward the end of the fetal period the vitreous portion of the hyaloid artery degenerates. The remaining part of the artery is then termed the *central artery of the retina.* In the adult, the former position of the vitreous portion of the hyaloid artery is indicated by the *hyaloid canal,* a minute passage extending through the vitreous body from the lens to the optic disc.

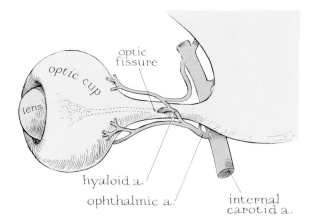

Stage 19 7th week (143)
Ventral view of the eye and the hyaloid artery about the end of the seventh week

Table 10. Components of the Eye and Their Embryonic Origins (173, 176)

Retina	Pars optica	Pigmented layer	Neural ectoderm (optic cup)
		Nervous layer	
	Pars caeca	Pars ciliaris retinae (contributes to ciliary body)	
		Pars iridica retinae (contributes to iris)	
Lens			Surface ectoderm
Sclera			Mesenchyme
Cornea		Stroma	Mesenchyme
		Epithelium	Surface ectoderm
Choroid			Mesenchyme
Iris		*(pars iridica retinae)* Smooth muscle, pigmented epithelium	Neural ectoderm (optic cup)
		Stroma	Mesenchyme
Ciliary body		*(pars ciliaris retinae)* Epithelium	Neural ectoderm (optic cup)
		Stroma, ciliary muscle	Mesenchyme

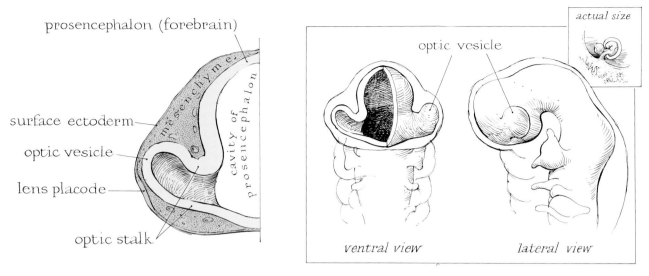

Figure 97. Stage 13
4–6 mm   28 days   4 weeks
(172)
Section of forebrain and optic vesicle

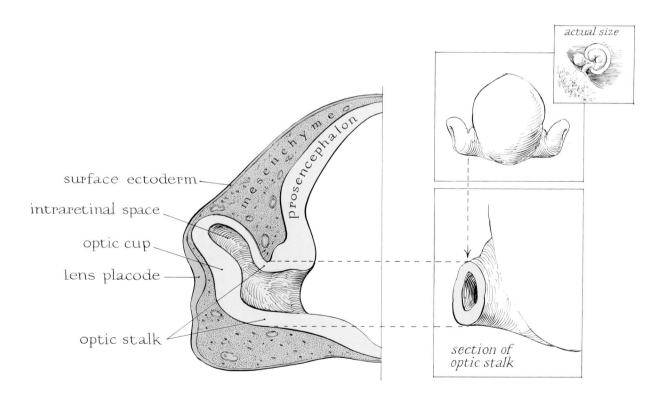

Figure 98. Stage 14
5–7 mm   32 days   5th week
(172)
Section of forebrain and optic cup

137

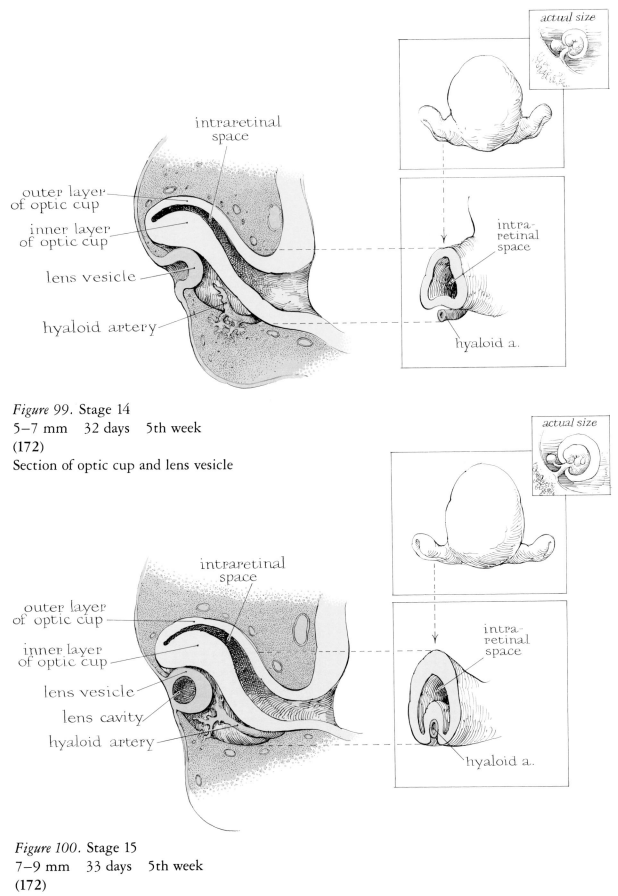

Figure 99. Stage 14
5–7 mm   32 days   5th week
(172)
Section of optic cup and lens vesicle

Figure 100. Stage 15
7–9 mm   33 days   5th week
(172)
Section of optic cup and lens vesicle

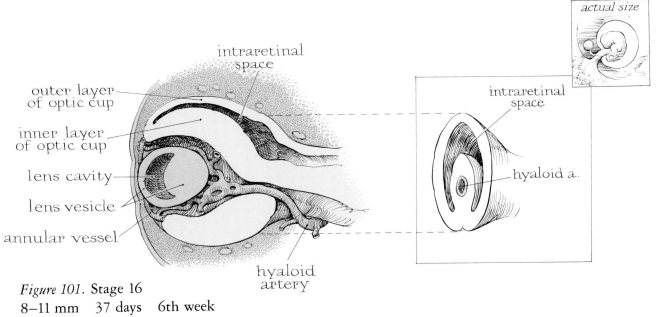

Figure 101. Stage 16
8–11 mm   37 days   6th week
(172, 177)
Section of optic cup and lens vesicle

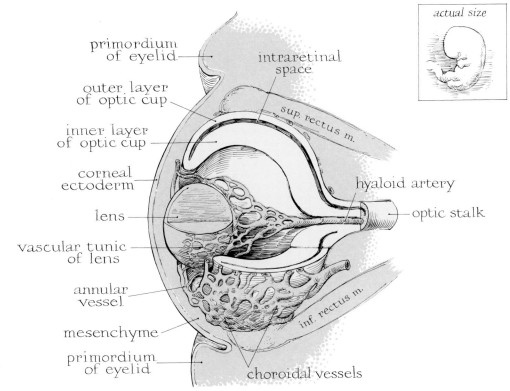

Figure 102. Stage 19
16–18 mm   48 days   7th week
(172, 175, 176, 177, 223)
Section of the eye

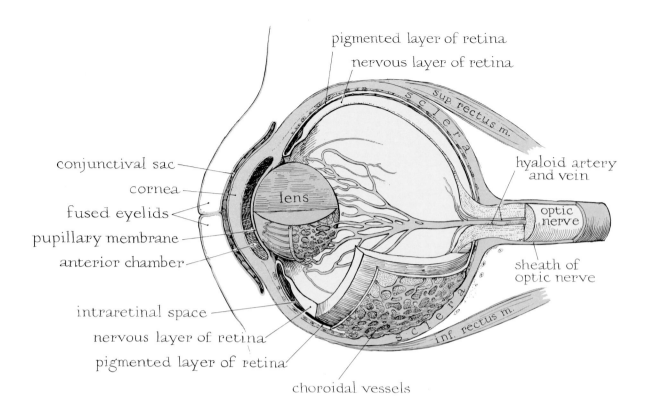

pigmented layer of retina

nervous layer of retina

sup. rectus m.

sclera

conjunctival sac

cornea

fused eyelids

pupillary membrane

anterior chamber

lens

hyaloid artery
and vein

optic
nerve

sheath of
optic nerve

intraretinal space

nervous layer of retina

pigmented layer of retina

sclera

inf. rectus m.

choroidal vessels

Figure 103. Early fetal period
50 mm   10 weeks
(5, 11, 172, 177)
Section of the eye

The Ear

The otic vesicle and the membranous labyrinth

Early in the fourth week the primordium of the inner ear can be identified dorsal to the second branchial groove as a thickened area of surface ectoderm termed the *otic placode*. During the fourth week the otic placode invaginates and separates from the ectoderm, forming a closed hollow structure termed the *otic vesicle*. Near the point of separation a new outgrowth, the *primordium of the endolymphatic sac,* develops on the medial aspect of the otic vesicle.

During the fifth and sixth weeks the ventral portion of the otic vesicle elongates, forming a curved tubular extension which is the *primordium of the cochlear duct.* The *primordia of the semicircular ducts* appear as three flanges extending from the dorsal aspect of the otic vesicle, and in the central portion of the vesicle paired evaginations foreshadow the development of the utricle and the saccule.

The primordia of the semicircular ducts are at first connected to the developing utricle by flattened areas of epithelium, but as the ducts grow in length, the central part of each area of epithelium becomes obliterated so that by the seventh week the three ducts stand free, connected to the utricle only at their ends.

As these changes occur, the utricle and the saccule become more clearly defined. The ventrally located saccule is connected to the cochlear duct, which continues to grow and coil until it reaches its final form of two and a half turns during the third month. All of these structures derived from the otic vesicle are collectively termed the *membranous labyrinth.* (See Figs. 104 and 105.)

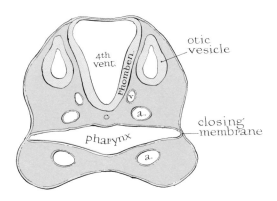

Stage 13   4 weeks (182, 186)
Coronal section of the head

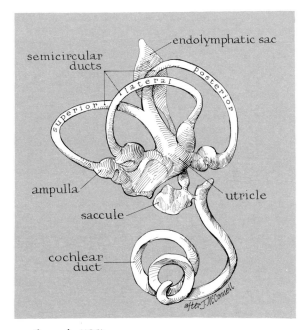

6 months (185)
Lateral view of the left membranous labyrinth

The osseous labyrinth

During the development of the membranous labyrinth the surrounding mesenchyme gives rise to the *cartilaginous otic capsule.* The cartilage immediately surrounding the membranous labyrinth subsequently undergoes resorption with the result that the membranous labyrinth comes to lie within a complex series of cavities termed the *cartilaginous labyrinth.*

The membranous labyrinth is filled with a clear fluid termed *endolymph* and is supported within the cartilaginous labyrinth by delicate strands of mesenchyme which extend between it and the surrounding cartilage. The cartilaginous labyrinth is filled with a clear fluid termed *perilymph.*

During the fifth month the cartilaginous otic capsule undergoes ossification and becomes the petrous part of the temporal bone. The space within which the membranous labyrinth lies is then termed the *osseous labyrinth.*

The cochlea and the spiral organ of Corti

Resorption of the cartilage around the cochlear duct results in the formation of two spaces, termed the *scala vestibuli* and the *scala tympani,* which are separated from each other by the *spiral lamina,* the *basilar membrane,* and the *cochlear duct.* Fibers of the cochlear nerve pass through the spiral lamina to reach sensory cells in the spiral organ of Corti.

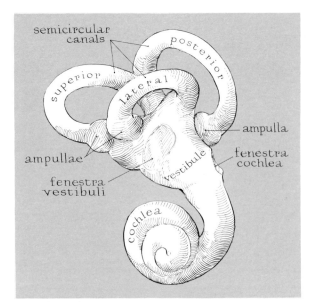

4 months (185, 187)
Lateral view of a cast of the left cartilaginous labyrinth. The space within the otic capsule has been filled with plastic and the surrounding cartilage has been removed.

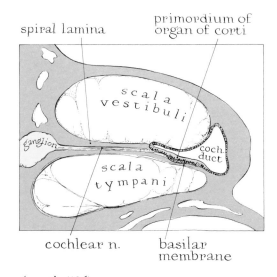

4 months (196)
Section through the second turn of the cochlea

142

The middle ear and the tympanic membrane

During the fourth week the endodermal lining of the first pharyngeal pouch makes contact with the ectodermal lining of the first branchial groove to form the *closing membrane*. This marks the site at which the tympanic membrane will develop. The first pharyngeal pouch will give rise to most of the auditory tube and the middle ear cavity, and the first branchial groove will become the external acoustic meatus.

During the fifth week the apposed layers of endoderm and ectoderm which form the closing membrane are invaded and separated by a broad wedge of mesenchyme. Within this mesenchyme the cartilaginous primordia of the auditory ossicles develop from the proximal portions of the first and second branchial arch cartilages.*

During the latter part of the fetal period an extension of the first pharyngeal pouch (the *tubotympanic recess*) grows around the auditory ossicles to form the tympanic cavity. A posterior expansion of the tympanic cavity forms the tympanic antrum and eventually the mastoid air cells. During this process the endodermal epithelium of the tympanic cavity envelopes the ossicles, which come to lie suspended within the tympanic cavity. The proximal part of the tubotympanic recess maintains its connection with the developing naso-pharynx and becomes the auditory tube.

*Some texts state that the first branchial cartilage forms the malleus and the incus, and that the second cartilage forms the stapes. However, analysis of the development of the auditory ossicles by Hanson (191) suggests that each auditory ossicle originates from more than one source.

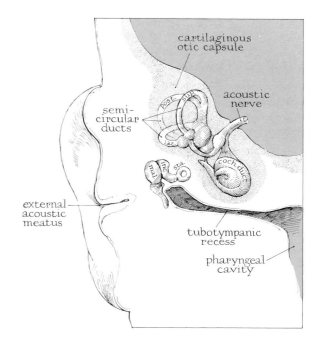

Late embryonic period (183, 191, 194)
Schematic coronal section of the ear about the end of the embryonic period. The cartilaginous otic capsule and the chondrocranium are represented as stippled areas.

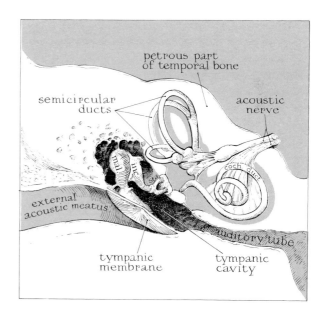

Newborn infant (23, 183, 189, 198)
Coronal section of the ear in the newborn infant

143

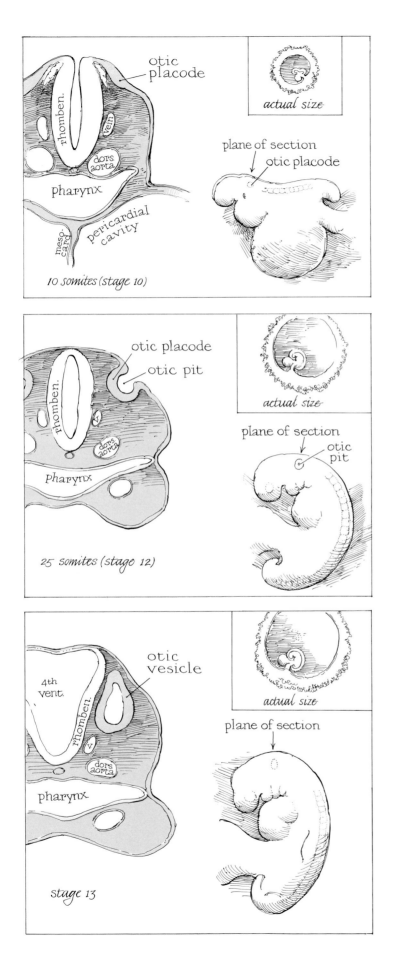

otic placode

rhomben.

vein

dors aorta

pharynx

meso card.

pericardial cavity

10 somites (stage 10)

plane of section
otic placode

actual size

otic placode

otic pit

rhomben.

dors aorta

Pharynx

25 somites (stage 12)

plane of section
otic pit

actual size

4th vent.

rhomben.

v.

dors aorta

otic vesicle

pharynx

stage 13

plane of section

actual size

Figure 104.
(30, 61, 182, 186, 192)
The development of the otic vesicle

Figure 105.
(194)
Development of the left membranous labyrinth (facing page)

c: cochlear nerve
cd: cochlear duct
cg: cochlear ganglion
cp: cochlear pouch
crus: common crus
endo duct: endolymphatic duct
endo sac: endolymphatic sac
lat sd: lateral semicircular duct
post sd: posterior semicircular duct
sac: saccule
sup sd: superior semicircular duct
ut: utricle
v: vestibular nerve
vg: vestibular ganglion
vp: vestibular pouch
VIII: acoustic nerve

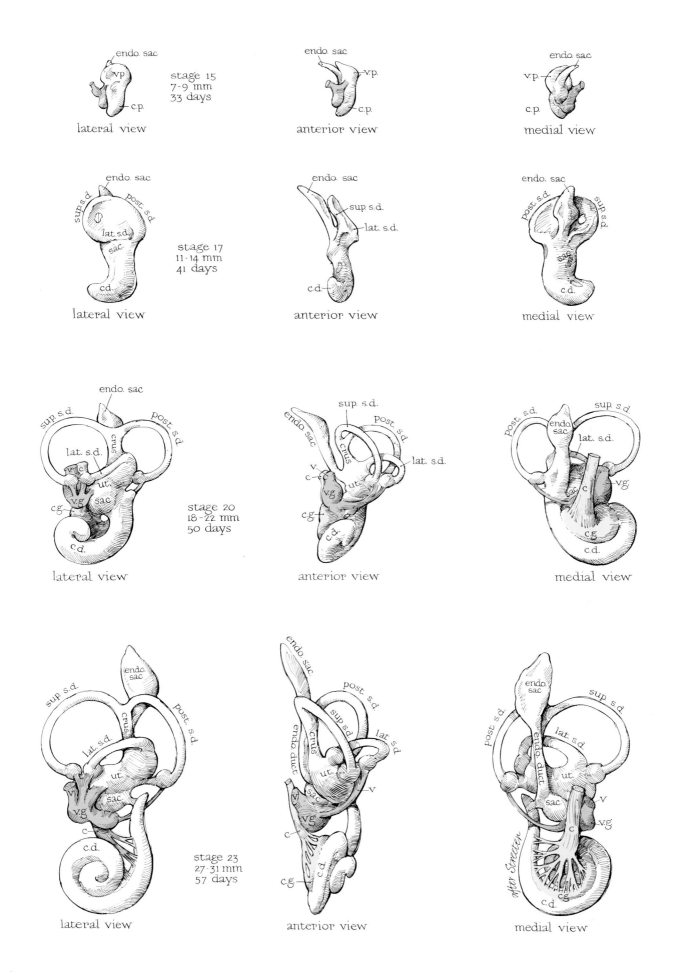

145

The Skeleton

Intramembranous and endochondral ossification

Bone development (ossification) takes place in two ways. In *intramembranous ossification* bone forms directly in mesenchyme. In *endochondral ossification* cartilage forms in mesenchyme. The cartilage subsequently undergoes resorption and is then replaced by bone.

It should be noted that this distinction is based solely on developmental criteria. The process of bone deposition is essentially the same in both cases, and in the adult there is no histological difference between bone which develops by endochondral ossification and bone which develops by intramembranous ossification.

All developing bones are surrounded by an osteogenic connective tissue membrane termed the *periosteum.* The flat bones of the skull grow by intramembranous ossification as the periosteum adds bone to the surface in successive layers. The long bones of the limbs grow in diameter by intramembranous ossification as the periosteum deposits a collar of bone around the shaft, but they grow in length by endochondral ossification at the epiphyseal plate.

With the exception of the clavicle, all bones of the trunk and limbs are preceded by miniature cartilaginous primordia which resemble the adult bone in shape. In a typical long bone the first, or primary center of ossification appears in the middle of the shaft of the cartilaginous primordium (the *diaphysis*) and progresses toward both ends (the *epiphyses*). Subsequently one or more secondary centers of ossification appear within each epiphysis. Between the epiphysis and the diaphysis there is a cartilaginous *epiphyseal plate* where growth in length occurs during childhood. At maturity the epiphyseal plate ossifies and no further bone growth is possible.

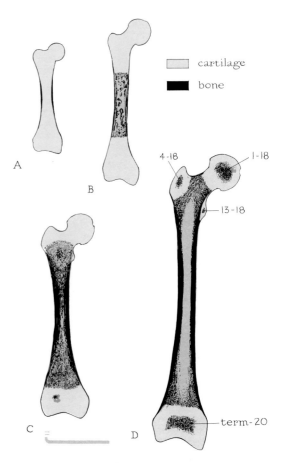

The progress of ossification as seen in longitudinal sections of the femur (205):

A. *Stage 22;* 8th week. A primary bony collar is laid down by intramembranous ossification.
B. *Ten weeks;* 55 mm. Endochondral ossification and formation of endochondral trabeculae occur in the middle of the shaft.
C. *Term.* Most of the shaft is ossified. The first center of epiphyseal ossification is seen in the distal extremity.
D. *Childhood.* Epiphyseal ossification centers are represented schematically. Numbers indicate the year of appearance and the year of fusion, respectively.

The vertebral column and ribs

Late in the fourth week mesenchymal cells of sclerotomal origin on either side of the notochord form the primordia of the vertebral bodies and disks. This occurs in such a way that the primordium of each vertebral body consists of contributions from two neighboring sclerotomes, and the primordium of each intervertebral disk lies opposite a myotome.

The notochord acts as an organizer during the development of the vertebral column but most of it undergoes resorption as the vertebral bodies form around it. Its only remnant persists as the *nucleus pulposus,* the soft core of the adult intervertebral disk.

Mesenchymal tissue derived from the vertebral primordia migrates dorsal and lateral to the neural tube to form the primordia of the neural arches and ribs. Like the vertebral bodies, the neural arches and ribs consist of contributions from adjacent sclerotomes.

During the seventh week centers of chondrification appear in the vertebral column. Ossification begins in the eighth week and continues throughout the fetal period and childhood, finally reaching its completion in young adulthood. The costal cartilages remain as the unossified part of the original cartilaginous costal elements.

The contribution of the neural crest

Most bone and cartilage is derived from the mesodermal germ layer, but certain bones and cartilages of the skull are now thought to be derived from the cranial part of the neural crest and therefore originally from neural ectoderm. This includes most of the branchial arch cartilages and their derivatives and possibly also portions of certain bones of the skull.

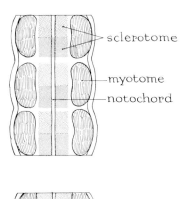

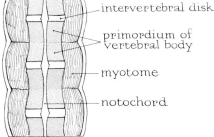

Schematic coronal section through the myotomes and the sclerotomes

Top: *Stage 13*   4 weeks
Bottom: *Stages 15 and 16*   5th week
The cranial and caudal portions of adjacent sclerotomes fuse to form the primordia of the vertebral bodies.

The chondrocranium

During the seventh week a number of separate cartilages develop around the base of the brain. These cartilages fuse to form an irregular cup-shaped structure termed the *chondrocranium*, which is subsequently replaced by bone.

The ethmoid bone develops from centers of ossification within the chondrocranium. It is the only skull bone which is entirely of endochondral origin. The sphenoid, temporal, and occipital bones develop as the result of the fusion of endochondral centers of ossification in the chondrocranium with intramembranous centers of ossification in the adjacent cranial mesenchyme.

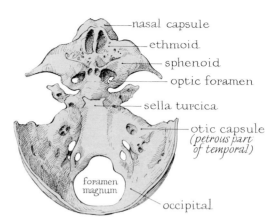

9th week   *40 mm* (212)
The interior of the chondrocranium

The branchial cartilages and their derivatives

The *branchial cartilages* are rod-like structures which develop within the branchial arches. The first branchial cartilage consists of dorsal and ventral parts around which the bones of the upper and lower jaws form. Most of the cartilage later undergoes resorption, except for small proximal portions which form most of the malleus and the incus.

The sphenomandibular ligament and probably a small part of the mandible in the region of the symphysis are also derived from the ventral part of the first (mandibular) arch. The second branchial cartilage makes a small contribution to the malleus and the incus. It also gives rise to most of the stapes, the styloid process, the stylohyoid ligament, and the upper part of the hyoid bone. The lower part of the hyoid bone arises from the third branchial cartilage. The fourth, fifth, and sixth branchial cartilages become the cartilages of the larynx.*

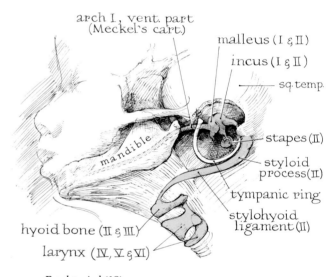

Fetal period (18)
The principal derivatives of the branchial arch cartilages are illustrated in a schematic lateral view of the head.

*Hanson (191).

148

Skull bones of intramembranous origin

Most of the vault of the skull is formed by the frontal and the parietal bones, which develop by intramembranous ossification. During the fetal period they are separated by unossified membranous sutures and fontanelles which allow for the growth of the brain and for the compression of the head during birth. The fontanelles close by the end of the second year, but complete closure of the sutures does not occur until adulthood.

Most of the bones of the face also develop by intramembranous ossification. The maxilla, the zygomatic, the palatine, and the vomer develop around the dorsal part of the first branchial cartilage, while the mandible develops around its ventral part.

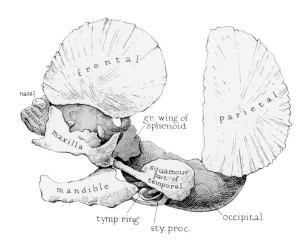

13 weeks   90 mm (12)
The principal bones of intramembranous origin as seen in a lateral view of the skull

The appendicular skeleton

The cartilaginous primordia of the appendicular skeleton originate from local mesenchyme in the limb buds. During the fifth week the pectoral and pelvic girdles begin to form, and development proceeds in a distal direction with the growth of the arms somewhat preceding that of the legs.

During the eighth week primary centers of ossification appear in the shafts of the long bones. Ossification continues throughout the fetal period, and at birth primary centers of ossification are found in all the limb bones except the patella, the carpals, and certain tarsals.

About the end of the fetal period secondary centers of ossification begin to appear in some of the epiphyses, and additional epiphyseal centers continue to develop during childhood and early adolescence. In late adolescence the epiphyses and the diaphyses fuse, and bone growth is complete.

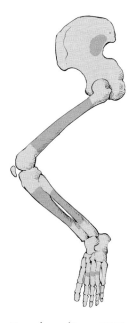

9 weeks   40 mm (221)
The cartilaginous primordia of the bones of the leg

149

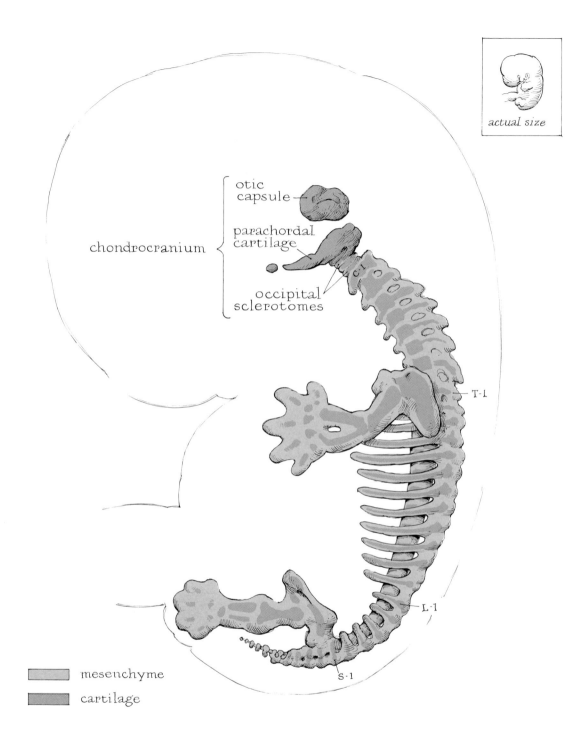

actual size

chondrocranium {
otic capsule
parachordal cartilage
occipital sclerotomes

C-1

T-1

L-1

S-1

mesenchyme
cartilage

Figure 106. Stage 18
13–17 mm   44 days   7th week
(2, 4, 11, 199, 200, 201, 203, 209)
Mesenchymal and cartilaginous skeletal
primordia. Left lateral view.

C-1: primordium of first cervical vertebra
T-1: primordium of first thoracic vertebra
L-1: primordium of first lumbar vertebra
S-1: primordium of first sacral vertebra

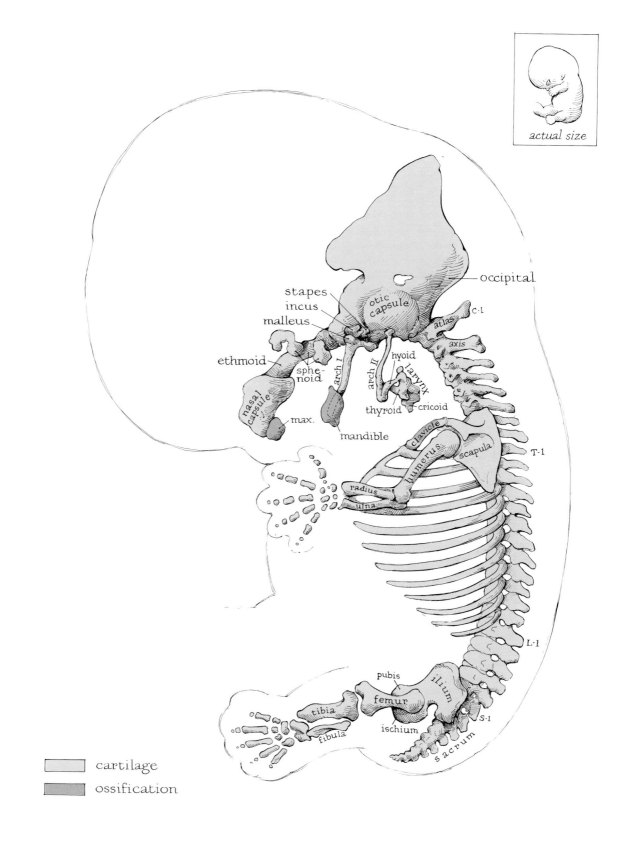

actual size

Figure 107. Stage 20
18–22 mm   50 days   8th week
(199, 200, 203, 204, 205, 209, 210, 216)

arch I: first branchial arch
arch II: second branchial arch
max: primordium of maxilla

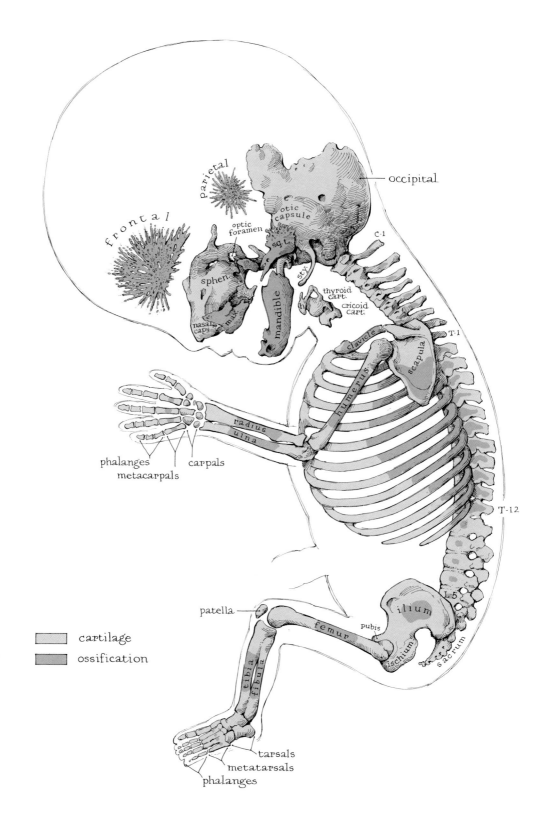

Figure 108. Early fetal period
40 mm   9 weeks
(4, 199, 200, 209, 211, 212)

h: hyoid
max: maxilla
sphen: sphenoid
sq t: squamous part of temporal bone
sty: styloid process

The Muscles

Smooth and cardiac muscle

Cardiac muscle and most of the smooth musculature are derived from splanchnic mesoderm. In some cases, however, smooth muscle originates from other sources. For instance, the smooth musculature of most blood vessels arises from adjacent mesenchyme, and the smooth muscles of the iris are thought to be derived from the neural ectoderm at the periphery of the optic cup. All the smooth and cardiac musculature is innervated by the autonomic nervous system.

The myotomes and their derivatives: the skeletal or voluntary muscles

About the beginning of the sixth week the myotomes differentiate into dorsal, or *epaxial* parts, and ventral, or *hypaxial* parts. Each myotome is innervated by a spinal nerve which gives a branch termed the *dorsal primary division* to the epaxial part and a *ventral primary division* to the hypaxial part. The epaxial parts of the myotomes develop into the extensor muscles of the dorsal part of the neck and trunk.

The fate of the hypaxial parts of the myotomes varies at different segmental levels. In the cervical region they form the infrahyoid musculature. In the thoracic and upper lumbar regions they form the intercostal musculature and the muscles of the abdominal wall. In the lower lumbar region they form the psoas and the quadratus lumborum muscles. In the sacral and coccygeal regions they form the musculature of the pelvic diaphragm.

The limb muscles are believed to originate from cells which migrate from somites adjacent to the limb buds. The tendons of these muscles, however, appear to develop from regional mesenchyme.

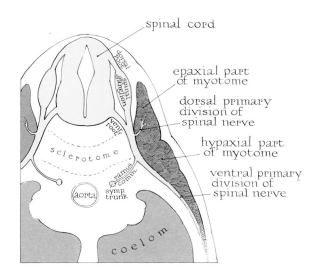

Stage 16 6th week (221)
Transverse section through the spinal cord and adjacent structures in the midthoracic region

153

Muscles of the head and neck

The eye muscles differentiate from a single mesenchymal condensation dorsal to the optic cup. The evidence of comparative anatomy suggests that they have evolved from three pro-otic myotomes (i.e., myotomes anterior to the otic capsule), but these myotomes have not been distinguished as separate entities in human embryos.

The muscles of mastication, the muscles of facial expression, and the muscles of the pharynx and the larynx originate from mesenchyme in the branchial arches. (A list of the muscles derived from each arch is given in table VII.)

The sternomastoid and trapezius muscles originate from a mass of mesoderm which may be derived either from occipital myotomes or from branchial arch muscles. The muscles of the tongue are thought to be derived from the last three occipital myotomes.

The diaphragm

The muscular part of the diaphragm is derived at least in part from mesenchyme in the transverse septum and in the dorsal and lateral body walls. The fact that the diaphragm receives its motor and part of its sensory innervation from components of the third, fourth, and fifth cervical nerves has been cited as evidence to support the theory that myoblasts from the corresponding cervical somites contribute to the formation of the muscular part of the diaphragm.

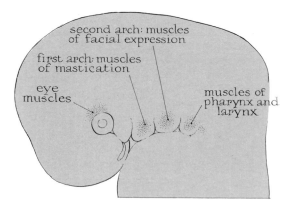

Stage 16 6th week
Lateral view of the head. Stippled areas indicate condensations of mesenchyme within the branchial arches.

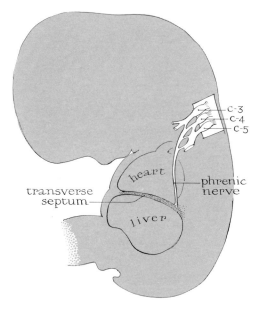

Stage 18 7th week
Lateral view of the phrenic nerve and the transverse septum. The muscular part of the diaphragm is beginning to develop within the transverse septum at this time.

Table 11. Origin and Innervation of the Visceral Arch Musculature (11)

Visceral Arch	Muscles	Nerves
1 Mandibular	Muscles of mastication (temporal, masseter, medial, and lateral pterygoids) Mylohyoid and anteriod belly of digastric Tensor palati and tensor pympani	V. Trigeminal—Mandibular division—(Post-trematic)
2 Hyoid	Facial group (including buccinator, extrinsic and intrinsic auricular muscles, occipito-frontalis, and platysma) Posterior belly of digastric and stylohyoid Stapedius	VII. Facial (Post-trematic)
3	Stylopharyngeus Probably part of upper pharyngeal muscles	IX. Glossopharyngeal (Post-trematic)
4, 5, and 6	Pharyngeal and laryngeal muscles	X. Vagus (superiod laryngeal and pharyngeal branches) (possibly XI)
	Laryngeal muscles	XI. Cranial fibers (possibly X) by way of the superior and recurrent laryngeal nerves
? post. 6	? Sternomastoid and trapezius	XI. (Spinal fibers)

155

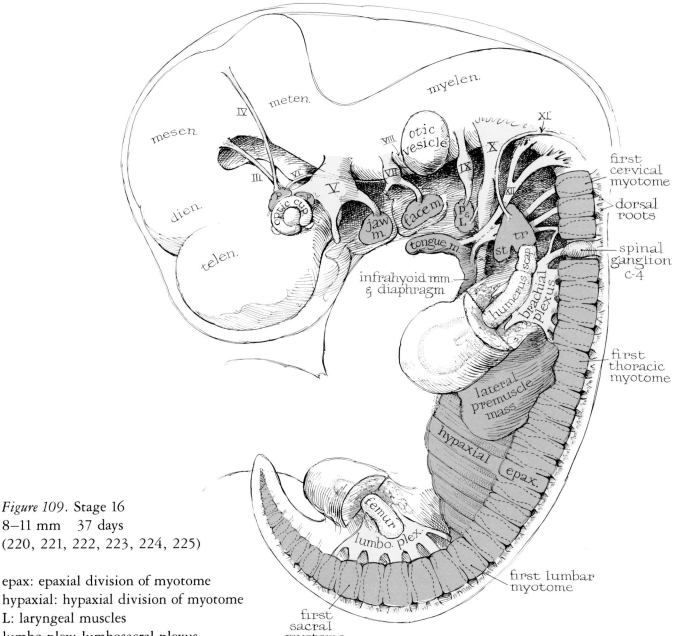

Figure 109. Stage 16
8–11 mm   37 days
(220, 221, 222, 223, 224, 225)

epax: epaxial division of myotome
hypaxial: hypaxial division of myotome
L: laryngeal muscles
lumbo plex: lumbosacral plexus
p: primordia of ocular muscles
scap: scapula
st: sternocleidomastoid
tr: trapezius
III: oculomotor nerve
IV: trochlear nerve
V: trigeminal ganglion nerve
VI: abducent nerve
VII: facial nerve
VIII: vestibulocochlear nerve
IX: glossopharyngeal nerve
X: vagus nerve
XI: accessory nerve
XII: hypoglossal nerve

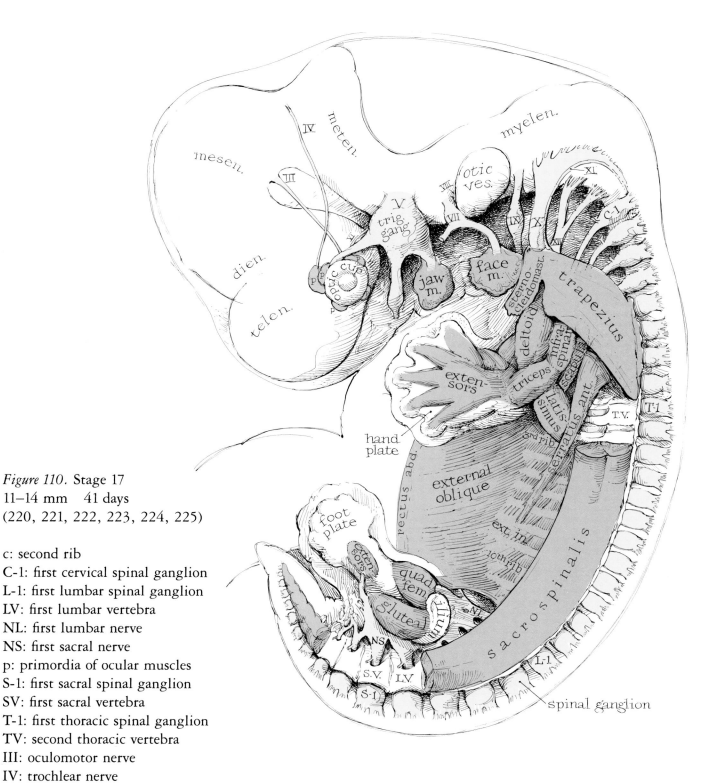

Figure 110. Stage 17
11–14 mm   41 days
(220, 221, 222, 223, 224, 225)

c: second rib
C-1: first cervical spinal ganglion
L-1: first lumbar spinal ganglion
LV: first lumbar vertebra
NL: first lumbar nerve
NS: first sacral nerve
p: primordia of ocular muscles
S-1: first sacral spinal ganglion
SV: first sacral vertebra
T-1: first thoracic spinal ganglion
TV: second thoracic vertebra
III: oculomotor nerve
IV: trochlear nerve
V: trigeminal nerve
VI: abducent nerve
VII: facial nerve
VIII: vestibulocochlear nerve
IX: glossopharyngeal nerve
X: vagus nerve
XI: accessory nerve
XII: hypoglossal nerve

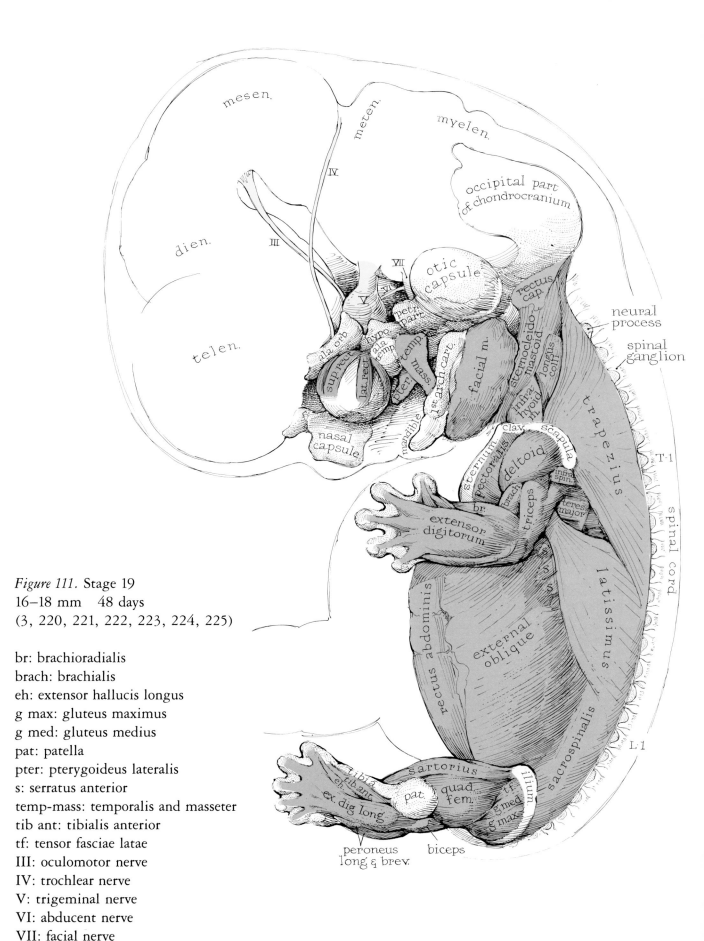

Figure 111. Stage 19
16–18 mm   48 days
(3, 220, 221, 222, 223, 224, 225)

br: brachioradialis
brach: brachialis
eh: extensor hallucis longus
g max: gluteus maximus
g med: gluteus medius
pat: patella
pter: pterygoideus lateralis
s: serratus anterior
temp-mass: temporalis and masseter
tib ant: tibialis anterior
tf: tensor fasciae latae
III: oculomotor nerve
IV: trochlear nerve
V: trigeminal nerve
VI: abducent nerve
VII: facial nerve

Appendix:
Comparable Stages in the Development of the Shark, Frog, Chick, and Human

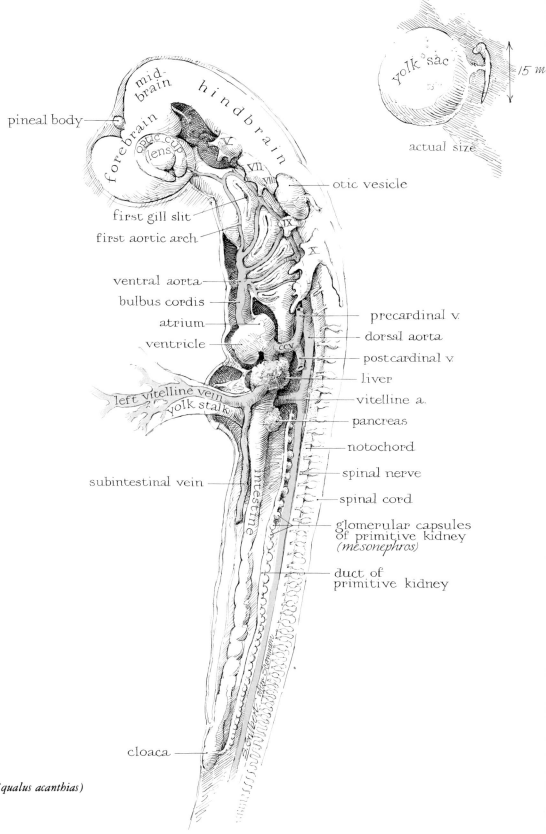

yolk sac

15 m

actual size

pineal body

mid-brain

hindbrain

forebrain

optic cup
(lens)

V

VII

VII

otic vesicle

IX

X

first gill slit

first aortic arch

ventral aorta

bulbus cordis

atrium

ventricle

CCV.

precardinal v.

dorsal aorta

postcardinal v.

liver

vitelline a.

pancreas

notochord

spinal nerve

spinal cord

glomerular capsules
of primitive kidney
(*mesonephros*)

duct of
primitive kidney

left vitelline vein

yolk stalk

subintestinal vein

intestine

cloaca

Figure 112. Shark embryo *(Squalus acanthias)*
of about 15 mm (20, 26)

V: trigeminal nerve
VIII: facial nerve
VIII: vestibulocochlear nerve
IX: glossopharyngeal nerve
X: vagus nerve

160

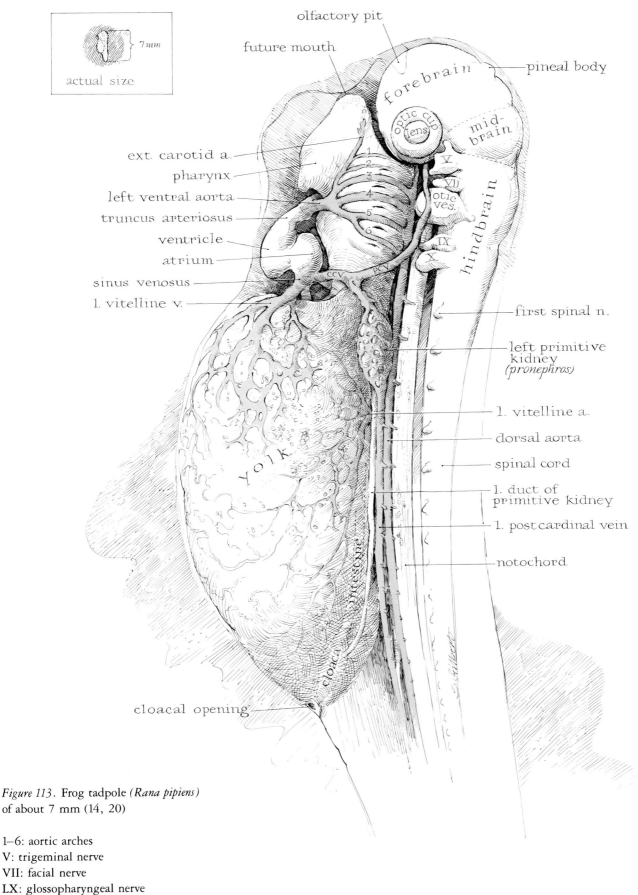

actual size

7 mm

olfactory pit

future mouth

pineal body

forebrain

optic cup

lens

mid-brain

ext. carotid a.

pharynx

left ventral aorta

truncus arteriosus

ventricle

atrium

sinus venosus

l. vitelline v.

V

VII

otic ves.

hindbrain

IX

X

CCV

PCV

yolk

cloaca

intestine

first spinal n.

left primitive kidney *(pronephros)*

l. vitelline a.

dorsal aorta

spinal cord

l. duct of primitive kidney

l. postcardinal vein

notochord

cloacal opening

Figure 113. Frog tadpole *(Rana pipiens)*
of about 7 mm (14, 20)

1–6: aortic arches
V: trigeminal nerve
VII: facial nerve
LX: glossopharyngeal nerve
X: vagus nerve

161

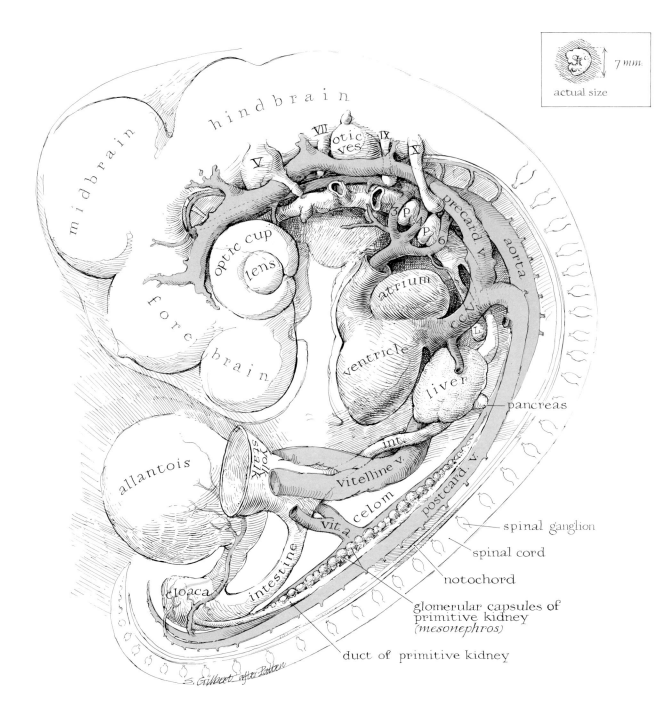

Figure 114. Chick embryo *(Gallus domesticus)*
of about 7 mm (4, 14, 25)

CCV: common cardinal vein
int: intestine
L: lung bud

P: pharyngeal pouch
V: trigeminal nerve
VII: facial nerve
IX: accessory nerve
XII: hypoglossal nerve

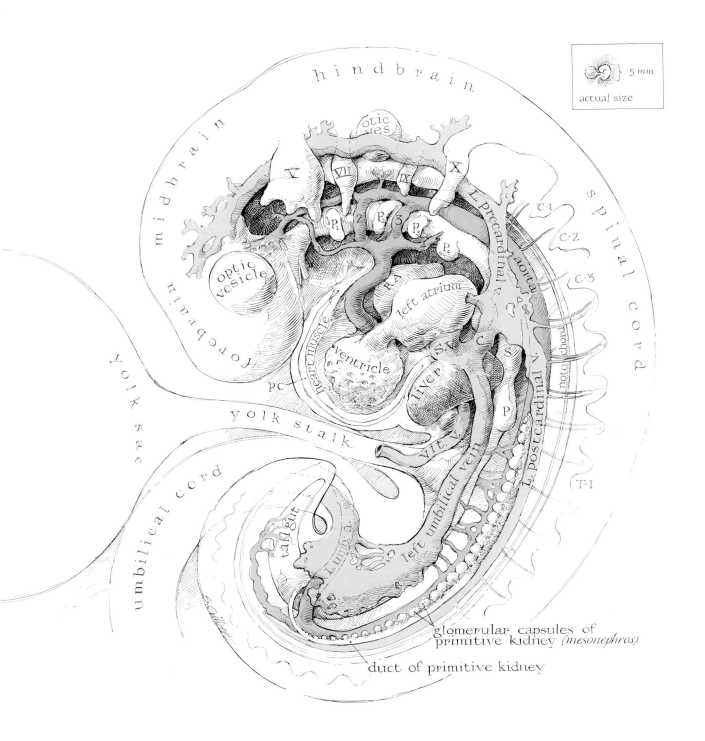

Figure 115. Human embryo
of about 5 mm (stage 13)
(61, 97, 115, 141, 143)

C: common cardinal vein
C-1: first cervical neural crest
P: dorsal pancreatic bud

RA: right atrium
S: stomach
SV: sinus venosus
T-1: first thoracic neural crest
vit. v: vitelline vein

Bibliography

Frequently cited journals have been identified by the following abbreviations:

Am. J. Anat.: American Journal of Anatomy
Anat. Rec.: The Anatomical Record
Carnegie Contrib. Embryol.: The Carnegie Institution of Washington Contributions to Embryology
J. Comp. Neurol.: Journal of Comparative Neurology
Z. Anat. Entwickl.-Gesch.: Zeitschrift für Anatomie und Entwicklungsgeschichte

TEXTS AND GENERAL WORKS

1. Arey, L. B. 1965. *Developmental anatomy.* 7th ed. Philadelphia: W. B. Saunders Co.
2. Blechschmidt, E. 1961. *The stages of human development before birth.* Philadelphia: W. B. Saunders Co.
3. ———. 1963. *The human embryo: Documentations on kinetic anatomy.* Stuttgart: Friedrich-Karl Schattauer Verlag.
4. Carlson, B. M. 1981. *Patten's foundations of embryology.* 4th ed. New York: McGraw-Hill Book Co.
5. Corliss, C. E. 1976. *Patten's human embryology: Elements of clinical development.* New York: McGraw-Hill Book Co.
6. Corning, H. K. 1925. *Lehrbuch der Entwicklungsgeschichte des Menschen.* Munich: J. F. Bergmann.
7. Crelin, E. S. 1969. *Anatomy of the newborn: An atlas.* Philadelphia: Lea and Febiger.
8. Gasser, R. F. 1975. *Atlas of human embryos.* New York: Harper and Row.
9. Gray, H. 1973. *Anatomy of the human body.* 29th American ed. Edited by C. M. Goss. Philadelphia: Lea and Febiger.
10. Gray, S. W. 1972. *Embryology for surgeons: The embryological basis for the treatment of congenital defects.* Philadelphia: W. B. Saunders Co.
11. Hamilton, W. J., and H. W. Mossman. 1972. *Human embryology.* 4th ed. Baltimore: The Williams and Wilkins Co.
12. Hertwig, O. 1915. *Die Elemente der Entwicklungsgeschichte des Menschen und der Wirbeltiere.* 5th ed. Jena: Verlag von Gustav Fischer.
13. His, W. 1885. *Anatomie menschlicher Embryonen.* 2 vols. Leipzig: F. C. W. Vogel.
14. Huettner, A. F. 1949. *Fundamentals of comparative embryology of the vertebrates.* 2d ed. New York: The Macmillan Co.
15. Jirasek, J. E. 1983. *Atlas of human prenatal morphogenesis.* Boston: Martinus Nijhoff.
16. Keibel, F., and F. P. Mall. 1910–12. *Manual of human embryology.* 2 vols. Philadelphia: J. B. Lippincott Co.
17. Kollman, J. 1898. *Lehrbuch der Entwicklungsgeschichte des Menschen.* Jena: Verlag von Gustav Fischer.
18. ———. 1907. *Handatlas der Entwicklungsgeschichte des Menschen.* 2 vols. Jena: Verlag von Gustav Fischer.
19. Kraus, B. S., H. Kitamura, and R. A. Latham. 1966. *Atlas of developmental anatomy of the face.* New York: Harper and Row.
20. Nelsen, O. E. 1953. *Comparative embryology of the vertebrates.* New York: The Blakiston Co.
21. Nishimura, H. 1977. *Prenatal development of the human with special reference to craniofacial structures: An atlas.* Bethesda, Md.: U.S. Dept. of Health, Education and Welfare Public Health Service.
22. O'Rahilly, R. 1975. *A color atlas of human embryology.* Philadelphia: W. B. Saunders Co.
23. Parke, W. W. 1975. *Photographic atlas of fetal anatomy.* Baltimore: University Park Press.
24. Patten, B. M. 1968. *Human embryology.* 3d ed. New York: McGraw-Hill Book Co.
25. ———. 1971. *Early embryology of the chick.* 5th ed. New York: McGraw-Hill Book Co.
26. Scammon, R. E. 1911. Normal plates of the development of *Squalus acanthias.* In Vol. 12 of *Normentafeln zur Entwicklungsgeschichte der Wirbeltiere,* edited by F. Keibel. Jena: Verlag von Gustav Fischer.

STUDIES OF INDIVIDUAL EMBRYOS

27. Atwell, W. J. 1930. A human embryo with 17 pairs of somites. *Carnegie Contrib. Embryol.* 21:1–24.
28. Brewer, J. 1938. A human embryo in the bilaminar blastodisc stage. *Carnegie Contrib. Embryol.* 27:85–93.

29. Bujard, E. 1914. Description d'un embryon humain, de 20 somites, avec flexion dorsale. *Internationale Monatsschrift für Anatomie und Physiologie* 31:238–66.

30. Corner, G. W. 1929. A well-preserved human embryo of 10 somites. *Carnegie Contrib. Embryol.* 20:81–102.

31. Dandy, W. E. 1910. A human embryo with seven pairs of somites measuring about 2 mm in length. *Am. J. Anat.* 10:85–108.

32. Davis, C. L. 1923. Description of a human embryo having twenty paired somites. *Carnegie Contrib. Embryol.* 15:1–51.

33. Elze, C. 1908. Beschreibung eines menschlichen Embryo von ca. 7 mm groesster Laenge. *Z. Anat. Entwickl.-Gesch.* 35:409–92.

34. Gage, S. P. 1905. A three weeks human embryo. *Am. J. Anat.* 4:409–43.

35. George, W. C. 1942. A presomite human embryo with chorda canal and prochordal plate. *Carnegie Contrib. Embryol.* 30:1–7.

36. Hertig, A. T., and J. Rock. 1941. Two human ova of the previllous stage, having an ovulation age of about eleven and twelve days respectively. *Carnegie Contrib. Embryol.* 29:127–56.

37. ———. 1945. Two human ova of the previllous stage, having a developmental age of about seven and nine days respectively. *Carnegie Contrib. Embryol.* 31:65–84.

38. ———. 1949. Two human ova of the previllous stage, having a developmental age of about eight and nine days respectively. *Carnegie Contrib. Embryol.* 33:169–86.

39. Hertig, A. T., et al. 1956. A description of 34 human ova within the first 17 days of development. *Am. J. Anat.* 98:435–93.

40. Heuser, C. H. 1930. A human embryo with 14 pairs of somites. *Carnegie Contrib. Embryol.* 22:135–53.

41. Heuser, C. H. 1932. A presomite human embryo with a definite chorda canal. *Carnegie Contrib. Embryol.* 23:251–67.

42. Heuser, C. H., et al. 1945. Two human embryos showing early stages of the definitive yolk sac. *Carnegie Contrib. Embryol.* 3:85–99.

43. Ingalls, N. W. 1907. Beschreibung eines menschlichen Embryos von 4.9 mm. *Archiv für mikroskopische Anatomie und Entwicklungsmechanik* 70:506–76.

44. ———. 1918. A human embryo before the appearance of the myotomes. *Carnegie Contrib. Embryol.* 7:111–34.

45. ———. 1920. A human embryo at the beginning of segmentation, with special reference to the vascular system. *Carnegie Contrib. Embryol.* 11:61–90.

46. Johnson, F. P. 1917. A human embryo of twenty-four pairs of somites. *Carnegie Contrib. Embryol.* 6:125–68.

47. Jones, H. O., and J. Brewer. 1911. A human embryo in the primitive streak stage (Jones-Brewer ovum I). *Carnegie Contrib. Embryol.* 29:157–65.

48. Krafka, J., Jr. 1941. The Torpin ovum, a presomite human embryo. *Carnegie Contrib. Embryol.* 29:167–93.

49. Ludwig, E. 1928. Ueber einen operativ gewonnenen menschlichen Embryo mit einem Ursegmente. *Gegenbaurs morphologisches Jahrbuch* 59:41–104.

50. ———. 1929. Embryon humain avec dix paires de somites mesoblastiques. *Comptes rendus de l'Association des Anatomistes* 24:580–85.

51. Payne F. 1925. General description of a 7-somite human embryo. *Carnegie Contrib. Embryol.* 16:115–24.

52. Piper, H. 1900. Ein menschlicher Embryo von 6.8 mm. *Archiv für Anatomie und Physiologie* [1900]:95–132.

53. Politzer, G. 1928. Ueber einen menschlichen Embryo mit 18 Ursegmentpaaren. *Z. Anat. Entwickl.-Gesch.* 87:674–727.

54. ———. 1930. Ueber einen menschlichen Embryo mit 7 Ursegmentpaaren. *Z. Anat. Entwickl.-Gesch.* 93:386–428.

55. Ramsey, E. M. 1937. The Lockyer embryo: An early human embryo *in situ. Carnegie Contrib. Embryol.* 26:99–119.

56. Rosenbauer, K. 1955. Untersuchung eines menschlichen Embryos mit 24 Somiten, unter besonderer Beruecksichtigung des Blutegefaess Systems. *Z. Anat. Entwickl.-Gesch.* 118:236–76.

57. Shaner, R. F. 1945. A human embryo of two to three pairs of somites. *Canadian Journal of Research* 23:235–43.

58. Sternberg, H. 1926. Beschreibung eines menschlichen Embryo mit vier Ursegmentpaaren, nebst Bemerkungen ueber die Anlage und Frueheste Entwicklung einiger Organe beim Menschen. *Z. Anat. Entwickl.-Gesch.* 82:142–240.

59. Steeter, G. L. 1920. A human embryo (Mateer) of the presomite period. *Carnegie Contrib. Embryol.* 9:389–424.

60. ———. 1942. Developmental horizons in human embryos. Description of age group XI, 13 to 20 somites, and age group XII, 21 to 29 somites. *Carnegie Contrib. Embryol.* 30:211–45.

61. ———. 1945. Developmental horizons in human embryos. Description of age group XIII, embryos about 4 or 5 millimeters long, and age group XIV, period of indentation of the lens vesicle. *Carnegie Contrib. Embryol.* 31:27–63.

62. ———. 1945. Developmental horizons in human embryos. Descriptions of age groups XV, XVI, XVII, and XVIII, being the third issue of a survey of the Carnegie Collection. *Carnegie Contrib. Embryol.* 32:133–203.

63. ———. 1951. Developmental horizons in human embryos. Descriptions of age groups XIX, XX, XXI, XXII, and XXIII, being the fifth issue of a survey of the Carnegie Collection. *Carnegie Contrib. Embryol.* 34:165–96.

64. Streiter, A. 1950. Ein menschlicher Keimling mit 7 Urwirbelpaaren. *Zeitschrift für mikroscopische-anatomische Forschung* 57:181–248.

65. Thompson, P. 1907. Description of a human embryo of 23 paired somites. *Journal of Anatomy and Physiology* 41:159–75.

66. Thyng, F. W. 1914. Anatomy of a 17.8 mm human embryo. *Am. J. Anat.* 17:31–112.

67. Viet, O. 1922. Untersuchung eines menschlichen Eies der vierten Woche. *Z. Anat. Entwickl.-Gesch.* 63:343–414.

68. Viet, O., and P. Esch. 1922. Untersuchung eines *in situ* fixierten, operative gewonnen menschlichen Eies der vierten Woche. *Archiv für Anatomie und Entwicklungs-geschichte* 63:243–414.

69. Wen, I. C. 1928. The anatomy of human embryos with seventeen to twenty-three pairs of somites. *J. Comp. Neurol.* 45:301–59.

70. West, C. M. 1930. Description of a human embryo of 8 somites. *Carnegie Contrib. Embryol.* 21:25–35.

71. Wilson, K. M. 1945. A normal human ovum of sixteen days development (the Rochester ovum). *Carnegie Contrib. Embryol.* 31:101–6.

EMBRYOS AND ILLUSTRATORS

72. Cullen, T. S. 1945. Max Broedel, 1870–1941, Director of the first department of art as applied to medicine in the world. *Bulletin of the Medical Library Association* 33:5–29.

73. Mall, F. P. 1904. Wilhelm His. *Am. J. Anat.* 4:139–61.

74. Waldeyer, W. 1904. Wilhelm His, sein Leben und Wirken. *Deutsche medizinische Wochenschrift* 39:1438–41; 40:1469–71; 41:1509–11.

THE FIRST THREE WEEKS

75. Bartelmez, G. W., and H. M. Evans. 1926. Development of the human embryo during the period of somite formation including embryos with 2 to 16 pairs of somites. *Carnegie Contrib. Embryol.* 17:1–67.

76. Boyd, J. D., and W. J. Hamilton. 1970. *The human placenta.* Cambridge: W. Heffer and Sons Ltd.

77. Chevallier, A., et al. Developmental fate of the somite mesoderm in the chick embryo. In *Vertebrate limb and somite morphogenesis,* edited by D. A. Ede, J. R. Hinchliffe, and Michael Balls. Cambridge: Cambridge University Press.

78. Hertig, A. T. 1968. *Human trophoblast.* Springfield, Ill.: Charles C. Thomas.

79. Luckett, W. P. 1978. Origin and differentiation of the yolk sac and extraembryonic mesoderm in presomite human and Rhesus monkey embryos. *Am. J. Anat.* 152:59–98.

80. McCrady, E., Jr. 1944. The evolution and significance of the germ layers. *Journal of the Tennessee Academy of Sciences* 19:240–51.

81. Oppenheimer, J. M. 1940. The non-specificity of the germ layers. *Quarterly Review of Biology* 15:1–27.

82. O'Rahilly, R. 1973. *Developmental stages in human embryos. Including a survey of the Carnegie Collection. Part A: Embryos of the first three weeks (stages 1 to 9).* Washington, D.C.: Carnegie Institute of Washington.

83. Ramsey, E., and M. W. Donner. 1980. *Placental vasculature and circulation.* Stuttgart: Georg Thieme.

THE DIGESTIVE AND RESPIRATORY SYSTEMS

84. Bardeen, C. R. 1914. The critical period in the development of the intestines. *Am. J. Anat.* 16:427–46.

85. Cullen, T. S. 1916. *Embryology, anatomy, and diseases of the umbilicus.* Philadelphia: W. B. Saunders Co.

86. Estrada, R. L. 1958. *Anomalies of intestinal rotation and fixation.* Springfield, Ill.: Charles C. Thomas.

87. Flint, J. M. 1906. The development of the lungs. *Am. J. Anat.* 6:1–138.

88. Fox, H. 1908. The pharyngeal pouches and their derivatives in the mammalia. *Am. J. Anat.* 8:187–250.

89. Frazer, J. E., and R. H. Robbins. 1915. On the factors concerned in causing rotation of the intestine in man. *Journal of Anatomy and Physiology* 50:75–110.

90. Heiss, R. 1919. Zur Entwicklung und Anatomie der menschlichen Lunge. *Archiv für Anatomie und Physiologie, Anatomische Abteilung* [1919]:1–129.

91. His, W. 1887. Zur Bildungsgeschichte der Lungen beim menschlichen Embryo. *Archiv für Anatomie und Physiologie, Anatomische Abteilung* [1887]:89–106.

92. Kingsbury, B. F. 1915. The development of the human pharynx. *Am. J. Anat.* 18:329–97.

93. Liu, H. M., and E. L. Potter. 1962. Development of the human pancreas. *Archives of Pathology* 74:439–52.

94. Mall, F. P. 1898. The development of the human intestine and its position in the adult. *Bulletin of the Johns Hopkins University Hospital* 9:197–208.

95. O'Rahilly, R. 1978. The timing and sequence of events in the development of the human digestive system and associated structures during the embryonic period proper. *Anatomy and Embryology* (Berlin) 153:123–36.

96. O'Rahilly, R., and E. A. Boyden. 1973. The timing and sequence of events in the development of the human respiratory system during the embryonic period proper. *Z. Anat. Entwickl.-Gesch.* 141:237–50.

97. Pernkopf, E. 1922–28. Die Entwicklung der Form des Magendarmkanals beim Menschen. *Z. Anat. Entwickl.-Gesch.* 64:96–275; 73:1–144; 77:1–143; 85:1–130.

98. Pohlmann, A. G. 1911. The development of the cloaca in human embryos. *Am. J. Anat.* 12:1–26.

99. Synder, W. H., Jr., and L. Chaffin. 1952. An intermediate stage in the return of the intestines from the umbilical cord (embryo 37 mm). *Anat. Rec.* 113:451–57.

100. Sudler, M. T. 1901. The development of the nose, and of the pharynx and its derivatives in man. *Am. J. Anat.* 1:391–415.

101. Tench, E. M. 1936. The development of the anus in the human embryo. *Am. J. Anat.* 59:333–45.

102. Thyng, F. W. 1908. Models of the pancreas in embryos of the pig, rabbit, cat, and man. *Am. J. Anat.* 7(4):489–503.

103. Weller, G. L. 1933. The development of the thyroid, parathyroid and thymus glands in man. *Carnegie Contrib. Embryol.* 24:93–139.

104. Wells, L. J., and E. Boyden. 1954. The development of the bronchopulmonary segments in human embryos of horizons XVII to XIX. *Am. J. Anat.* 95:163–201.

THE UROGENITAL SYSTEM

105. Gyllensten, L. 1949. Contributions to the embryology of the urinary bladder. Part 1: The development of the definitive relations between the openings of the Wolffian ducts and the ureters. *Acta Anatomica* 7(4):305–44.

106. Hill, E. C. 1907. On the gross development and vascularization of the testis. *Am. J. Anat.* 6:1–137.

107. Huber, C. G. 1904. On the development and shape of the uriniferous tubules of certain higher mammals. *Am. J. Anat.* 4(supp.):1–98.

108. Hunter, R. H. 1930. Observations on the development of the human female genital tract. *Carnegie Contrib. Embryol.* 22:91–108.

109. Kelley, H. A., and C. F. Burnam. 1922. *Diseases of the kidneys, ureters, and bladder. Vol. 1.* New York: D. Appleton-Century Co.

110. Koff, A. K. 1933. Development of the vagina in the human fetus. *Carnegie Contrib. Embryol.* 24:59–90.

111. Lowsey, O. S. 1912. The development of the human prostrate gland with reference to the development of other structures at the neck of the urinary bladder. *Am. J. Anat.* 13:299–349.

112. O'Rahilly, R. 1973. The embryology and anatomy of the uterus. In *International Academy of Pathology Monograph no. 14,* 17–39. Baltimore: The Williams and Wilkins Co.

113. O'Rahilly, R., and E. C. Muecke. 1972. The timing and sequence of events in the development of the human urinary system during the embryonic period proper. *Z. Anat. Entwickl.-Gesch.* 138(1):99–109.

114. Patten, B. M., and A. Barry. 1952. The genesis of exstrophy of the bladder and epispadias. *Am. J. Anat.* 90:35–57.

115. Shikinami, J. 1926. Detailed form of the Wolffian body in human embryos of the first eight weeks. *Carnegie Contrib. Embryol.* 18:49–62.

116. Spaulding, M. H. 1921. The development of the external genitalia in the human embryo. *Carnegie Contrib. Embryol.* 13:67–88.

117. Torrey, T. W. 1954. The early development of the human nephros. *Carnegie Contrib. Embryol.* 35:175–98.

118. ———. 1965. Morphogenesis of the vertebrate kidney. In *Organogenesis,* by DeHaan and Ursprung, 559–79. New York: Holt, Rinehart and Winston.

119. Witschi, E. 1948. Migration of the germ cells of human embryos from the yolk sac to the primitive gonadal folds. *Carnegie Contrib. Embryol.* 32:67–80.

THE HEART

120. Born, G. 1889. Beitraege zur Entwicklungsgeschichte des Saugethierherzens. *Archiv für mikroskopische Anatomie und Entwicklungsmechanik* 33:284–377.

121. Cooper, M., and R. O'Rahilly. 1971. The human heart at seven postovulatory weeks. *Acta Anatomica* 79:280–99.

122. Davis, C. L. 1927. Development of the human heart from its first appearance to the stage found in embryos of twenty paired somites. *Carnegie Contrib. Embryol.* 19:245–84.

123. De Vries, P. A., and J. B. de C. M. Saunders. 1962. Development of the ventricles and spiral outflow tract in the human heart. A contribution to the development of the human heart from age group IX to age group XV. *Carnegie Contrib. Embryol.* 37:87–114.

124. Goss, C. M. 1952. Development of the median coordinated ventricle from the lateral hearts in rat embryos with three to six somites. *Anat. Rec.* 112:761–96.

125. Kramer, T. C. 1942. The partitioning of the truncus and conus and the formation of the membranous portion of the interventricular septum in the human heart. *Am. J. Anat.* 71:343–70.

126. Licata, R. H. 1954. The human embryonic heart in the ninth week. *Am. J. Anat.* 94:73–126.

127. Mall, F. P. 1912. On the development of the human heart. *Am. J. Anat.* 13:249–98.

128. Odgers, P. N. B. 1935. The formation of the venous valves, the foramen secundum and the septum secundum in the human heart. *Journal of Anatomy* 69:412–22.

129. ———. 1938. The development of the pars membranacea septi in the human heart. *Journal of Anatomy* 72:247–59.

130. O'Rahilly, R. 1971. The timing and sequence of events in human cardiogenesis. *Acta Anatomica* 79:70–75.

131. Patten, B. M. 1960. Persistent interatrial foramen primum. *Am. J. Anat.* 107:217–80.

132. Patten, B. M., et al. 1929. Functional limitations of the foramen ovale in the human foetal heart. *Anat. Rec.* 44:165–78.

133. Tandler, J. 1912. The development of the heart. In *Manual of human embryology,* edited by F. Keibel and F. P. Mall, Vol. 2, 534–70. Philadelphia: J. B. Lippincott Co.

134. ———. 1913. Anatomie des Herzens. 3 Band, 1 Abt. In *Handbuch der Anatomie des Menschen,* edited by K. H. Bardeleben. Jena: Verlag von Gustave Fischer.

135. Vernall, D. G. 1962. The human embryonic heart in the seventh week. *Am. J. Anat.* 111:17–24.

136. Walls, E. W. 1947. The development of the specialized conducting tissue of the human heart. *Journal of Anatomy* 81:93–110.

137. Waterston, D. 1918. The development of the heart in man. *Royal Society of Edinburgh, Transactions* 52(pt. 2): 257–301.

THE ARTERIES

138. Barry, A. 1951. The aortic arch derivatives in the human adult. *Anat. Rec.* 111:221–38.

139. Bremer, J. L. 1909. On the origin of the pulmonary arteries in mammals. *Am. J. Anat.* 1:138–44.

140. ———. 1915. The origin of the renal artery in mammals and its anomalies. *Am. J. Anat.* 18:179–200.

141. Congdon, E. D. 1922. Transformation of the aortic arch system during the development of the human embryo. *Carnegie Contrib. Embryol.* 14:47–110.

142. Heuser, C. H., et al. 1923. The branchial vessels and their derivatives in the pig. *Carnegie Contrib. Embryol.* 15:121–39.

143. Padget, D. H. 1948. Development of the cranial arteries in the human embryo. *Carnegie Contrib. Embryol.* 32:205–61.

144. Senior, H. D. 1919. On the development of the arteries of the human lower extremity. *Am. J. Anat.* 25:55–95.

145. Streeter, G. L. 1918. Developmental alterations in the vascular system of the brain of the human embryo. *Carnegie Contrib. Embryol.* 8:5–38.

THE VEINS

146. Bremer, J. L. 1937. Two reconstructions explaining the development of the veins of the liver. *Anat. Rec.* 68:165–68.

147. Butler, E. G. 1927. The relative role played by the embryonic veins in the development of the mammalian vena cava posterior. *Am. J. Anat.* 39:267–353.

148. Gruenwald, P. 1938. Die Entwicklung der Vena cava Caudalis beim Menschen. *Zeitschrift für mikroscopische-anatomische Forschung* 43:275–331.

149. Mall, F. P. 1906. A study of the structural unit of the liver. *Am. J. Anat.* 5:227–308.

150. McClure, C. F., and E. G. Butler. 1925. The development of the vena cava inferior in man. *Am. J. Anat.* 35:331–83.

151. McClure, C. F., and G. S. Huntington. 1929. The mammalian vena cava posterior. *American Anatomical Memoirs* 15:[56 unnumbered pages].

152. Neill, C. A. 1956. Development of the pulmonary veins. *Pediatrics* 18:880–87.

153. Padget, D. H. 1956. The cranial venous system in man in reference to development, adult configuration, and relation to the arteries. *Am. J. Anat.* 98:307–56.

154. ———. 1957. The development of the cranial venous system in man, from the viewpoint of comparative anatomy. *Carnegie Contrib. Embryol.* 36:79–140.

155. Streeter, G. L. 1915. The development of the venous sinuses of the dura mater in the human embryo. *Am. J. Anat.* 18:145–78.

THE NERVOUS SYSTEM

156. Bartelmez, G. W., and A. S. Dekaban. 1962. The early development of the human brain. *Carnegie Contrib. Embryol.* 37:13–32.

157. Hines, M. 1922. Studies on the growth and differentiation of the telencephalon in man. *J. Comp. Neurol.* 34:73–171.

158. His, W. 1893. Vorschlaege zur Eintheilung des Gehirns. *Archiv für Anatomie und Entwicklungsgeschichte, Anatomische Abteilung* [1893]:172–79.

159. Hochstetter, F. 1929. *Beitraege zur Entwicklungsgeschichte des menschlichen Gehirns.* Vienna and Leipzig: Deuticke.

160. Kingsbury, B. F. 1920. The extent of the floor-plate and its significance. *J. Comp. Neurol.* 32:113–33.

161. ———. 1922. The fundamental plan of the vertebrate brain. *J. Comp. Neurol.* 34:461–86.

162. ———. 1930. The developmental significance of the floor-plate of the brain and spinal cord. *J. Comp. Neurol.* 50:177–201.

163. Lemire, R. 1975. *Normal and abnormal development of the human nervous system.* New York: Harper and Row.

164. O'Rahilly, R., and E. Gardner. 1971. The timing and sequence of events in the development of the human nervous system. *Z. Anat. Entwickl.-Gesch.* 134:1–12.

165. Pick, J. 1970. *The autonomic nervous system.* Philadelphia: J. B. Lippincott.

166. Sensenig, E. C. 1951. The early development of the meninges of the spinal cord in human embryos. *Carnegie Contrib. Embryol.* 34:145–57.

167. ———. 1957. The development of the occipital and cervical segments and their associated structures in human embryos. *Carnegie Contrib. Embryol.* 36:141–51.

168. Streeter, G. L. 1904. The development of the cranial and spinal nerves in the occipital region of the human embryo. *Am. J. Anat.* 4:83–116.

169. ———. 1908. The peripheral nervous system in the human embryo at the end of the first month (10 mm). *Am. J. Anat.* 8:285–301

170. ———. 1912. The development of the nervous system. In *Manual of human embryology*, edited by F. Keibel and F. P. Mall, Vol. 2, 1–156. Philadelphia: J. B. Lippincott.

171. Yntema, C. L., and W. S. Hammond. 1947. The development of the autonomic nervous system. *Biological Review* 22:344–59.

THE EYE

172. Bach, L., and R. Seefelder. 1914. *Atlas zur Entwicklungsgeschichte des menschlichen Auges.* Leipzig: Englemann.

173. Barber, A. N. 1955. *Embryology of the human eye.* St. Louis: The C. V. Mosby Co.

174. Dejean, C., et al. 1958. *L'embryologie de l'oeil et sa teratologie.* Paris: Masson.

175. Duke-Elder, S., and C. Cook. 1963. Normal and abnormal development. Part 1 in Vol. 3 of *System of ophthalmology,* edited by S. Duke-Elder. St. Louis: The C. V. Mosby Co.

176. Jacobiec, F. A. 1982. *Ocular anatomy, embryology, and teratology.* Philadelphia: Harper and Row.

177. Mann, I. 1957. *The development of the human eye.* 3d ed. New York: Grune and Stratton.

178. Morone, G., et al. 1981. *The vascular system of the eye.* Pavia: Edizione la Goliardica Pavese.

179. O'Rahilly, R. 1966. The early development of the eye in staged human embryos. *Carnegie Contrib. Embryol.* 38:1–42.

180. Weiss, P. A. 1950. Perspectives in the field of morphogenesis. *Quarterly Review of Biology* 25:177–98.

THE EAR

181. Anson, B. J., and T. H. Bast. 1946. The development of the auditory ossicles and associated structures in man. *Annals of Otology, Rhinology, and Laryngology* 55:467–94.

182. Anson, B. J., and W. T. Black. 1934. The early relation of the auditory vesicle to the ectoderm in human embryos. *Anat. Rec.* 58:127–37.

183. Anson, B. J., and J. A. Donaldson. 1981. *Surgical anatomy of the temporal bone.* 3d ed. Philadelphia: W. B. Saunders Co.

184. Anson, B. J., and J. Martin. 1938. Otic capsule and membranous labyrinth of the 29 mm (crown-rump) human embryo. *Archives of Otolaryngology* 27:279–303.

185. Anson, B. J., et al. 1967. The vestibular system: Anatomic considerations. *Archives of Otolaryngology* 85:497–514.

186. Bartelmez, G. W. 1922. The origin of the otic primordia in man. *J. Comp. Neurol.* 34:201–32.

187. Bast, T. H. 1930. Ossification of the otic capsule in human fetuses. *Carnegie Contrib. Embryol.* 21:53–82.

188. Bast, T. H., and W. D. Gardiner. 1947. The developmental course of the human auditory vesicle. *Anat. Rec.* 99:55–74.

189. Broedel, M. 1946. *Three unpublished drawings of the anatomy of the human ear.* Philadelphia: W. B. Saunders Co.

190. Hammar, J. A. 1902. Studien uber die Entwicklung des Vorderdarms und einiger angrenzender Organe. *Archiv für mikroskopische Anatomie und Entwicklungs-mechanik* 59:471–628.

191. Hanson, J. R., B. J. Anson, and E. M. Strickland. 1962. Branchial sources of the auditory ossicles in man. Part 2. Observations of embryonic stages from 7 mm to 28 mm (CR length). *Archives of Otolaryngology* 76:200–215.

192. O'Rahilly, R. 1963. The early development of the otic vesicle in staged embryos. *Journal of Embryology and Experimental Morphology* 11:741–55.

193. Siebenmann, F. 1922. Ein neues Labyrinth-modell des menschlichen Gehoerorganes. *Zeitschrift für Ohrenheilkunde* 82:1–4.

194. Streeter, G. L. 1907. On the development of the membranous labyrinth and the acoustic and facial nerves in the human embryo. *Am. J. Anat.* 6:139–66.

195. ———. 1917. The development of the scala tympani, scala vestibuli and perioticular cistern in the human embryo. *Am. J. Anat.* 21:299–320.

196. ———. 1918. The histogenesis and growth of the otic capsule and its contained periotic tissue-spaces in the human embryo. *Carnegie Contrib. Embryol.* 7:5–54.

197. Strickland, E. M., et al. 1962. Branchial sources of the auditory ossicles in man. Part 1. *Archives of Otolaryngology* 76:101–22.

198. Wong, M. L. 1983. Embryology and developmental anatomy of the ear. Pages 85–111 in Vol. 1 of *Pediatric otolaryngology*, edited by C. D. Bluestone and S. E. Stool. Philadelphia: W. B. Saunders.

THE SKELETON

199. Bardeen, C. R. 1905. The development of the thoracic vertebrae in man. *Am. J. Anat.* 4:163–74.

200. ———. 1905. Studies on the development of the human skeleton. *Am. J. Anat.* 4:265–302.

201. ———. 1908. Early development of the cervical vertebrae and the base of the occipital bone in man. *Am. J. Anat.* 8:181–86.

202. Breathnach, A. S., editor. 1965. *Frazer's anatomy of the human skeleton*. 6th ed. Boston: Little, Brown and Co.

203. De Beer, G. R. 1937. *The development of the vertebrate skull*. London: Oxford University Press.

204. Fawcett, E. 1910. Description of a reconstruction of the head of a thirty-millimeter embryo. *Journal of Anatomy* 44:303–11.

205. Gardner, E., and D. J. Gray. 1970. The prenatal development of the human femur. *Am. J. Anat.* 129:121–40.

206. Graefenberg, E. 1906. Die Entwicklung der Knochen, Muskeln, und Nerven der Hand. *Z. Anat. Entwickl.-Gesch.* (Anat. Hefte) 30:1–154.

207. Kernan, J. D. 1916. The chondrocranium of a 20 mm human embryo. *Journal of Morphology* 27:605–46.

208. Levi, G. 1900. Beitrag zum Studium der Entwicklung des knorpeligen Primordialcraniums des Menschen. *Archiv für mikroskopische Anatomie und Entwicklungs-mechanik* 55:341–414.

209. Lewis, W. H. 1902. The development of the arm in man. *Am. J. Anat.* 1:145–83.

210. Lewis, W. H. 1920. The cartilaginous skull of a human embryo 21 mm in length. *Carnegie Contrib. Embryol.* 9:299–324.

211. Macklin, C. C. 1914. The skull of a human foetus of 40 mm. *Am. J. Anat.* 16:317–426.

212. ———. 1921. The skull of a human fetus of 43 mm greatest length. *Carnegie Contrib. Embryol.* 10:57–103.

213. Noback, C. R. 1944. The developmental anatomy of the human osseous skeleton during the embryonic, fetal, and circumnatal periods. *Anat. Rec.* 88:91–125.

214. Noback, C. R., and G. G. Robertson. 1951. Sequences of the appearance of ossification centers in the human skeleton during the first five prenatal months. *Am. J. Anat.* 89:1–28.

215. Olivier, G. 1962. *Formation du squelette des membres*. Paris: Vigot Frères.

216. O'Rahilly, R., and E. Gardiner. 1972. The initial appearance of ossification in staged human embryos. *Am. J. Anat.* 134:291–307.

217. Sensenig, E. C. 1949. The early development of the human vertebral column. *Carnegie Contrib. Embryol.* 33:21–41.

218. Streeter, G. L. 1949. Developmental horizons in human embryos. A review of the histogenesis of cartilage and bone. *Carnegie Contrib. Embryol.* 33(4):149–67.

219. Youssef, E. H. 1964. The development of the skull in a 34 mm human embryo. *Acta Anatomica* 57:72–90.

THE MUSCLES

220. Bardeen, C. R. 1907. Development and variation of the nerves and the musculature of the inferior extremity and the neighbouring regions of the trunk in man. *Am. J. Anat.* 6:259–390.

221. Bardeen, C. R., and W. H. Lewis. 1901. Development of the limbs, body wall, and back in man. *Am. J. Anat.* 1:1–37.

222. Gasser, R. F. 1967. Development of the facial muscles in man. *Am. J. Anat.* 120:357–76.

223. Gilbert, P. W. 1957. The origin and development of the human extrinsic ocular musculature. *Carnegie Contrib. Embryol.* 36:59–78.

224. Lewis, W. H. 1901. The development of the arm in man. *Am. J. Anat.* 1:145–84.

225. McKenzie, J. 1962. The development of the sternomastoid and trapezius muscles. *Carnegie Contrib. Embryol.* 37:123–29.

226. Wells, L. J. 1954. Development of the human diaphragm and pleural sacs. *Carnegie Contrib. Embryol.* 35:107–34.

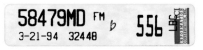